Endometriosis - Recent Advances, New Perspectives and Treatments

Edited by Giovana Ap. Gonçalves

Published in London, United Kingdom

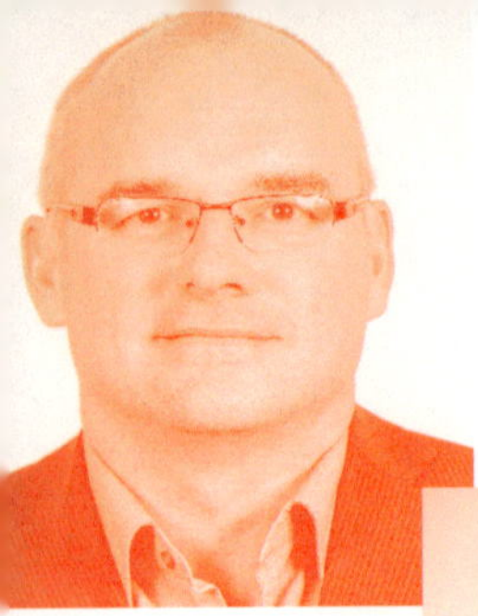

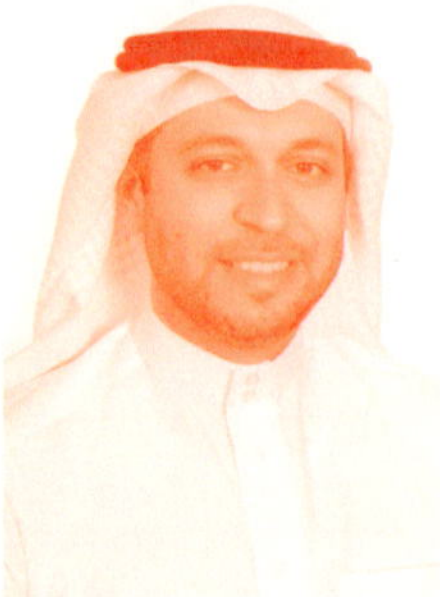

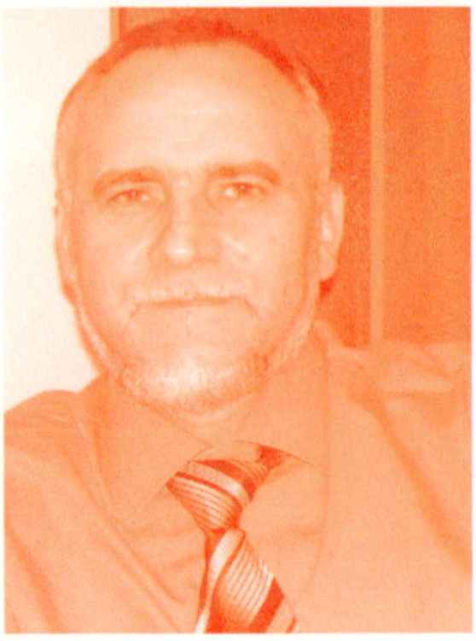

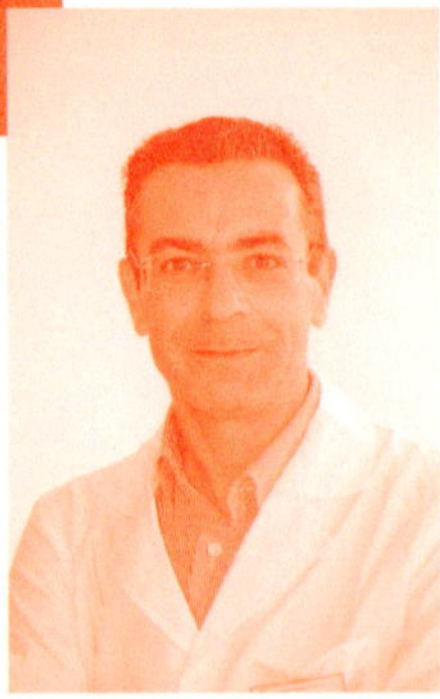

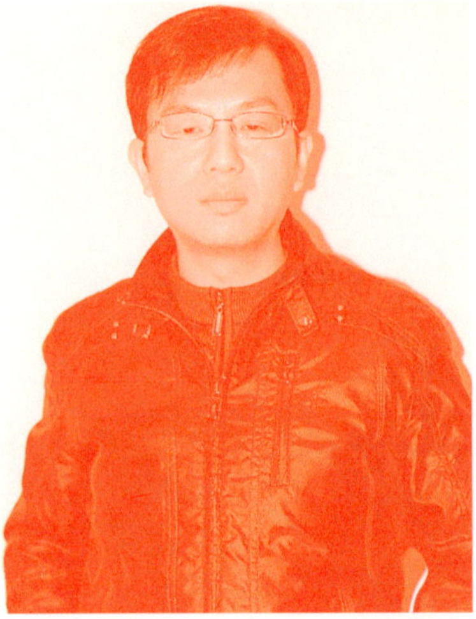

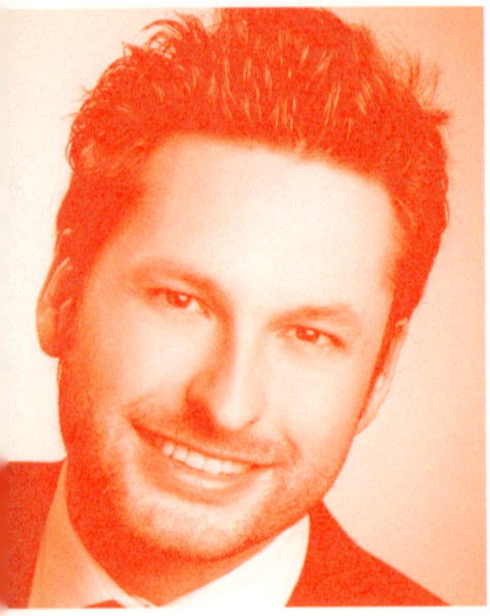

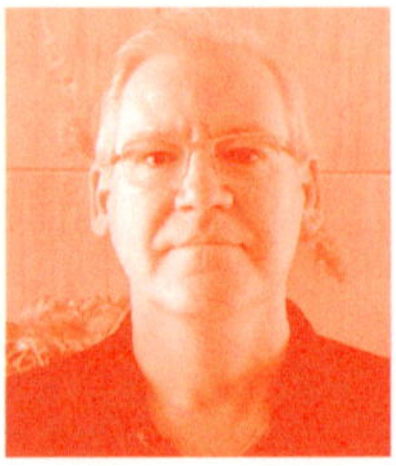

IntechOpen

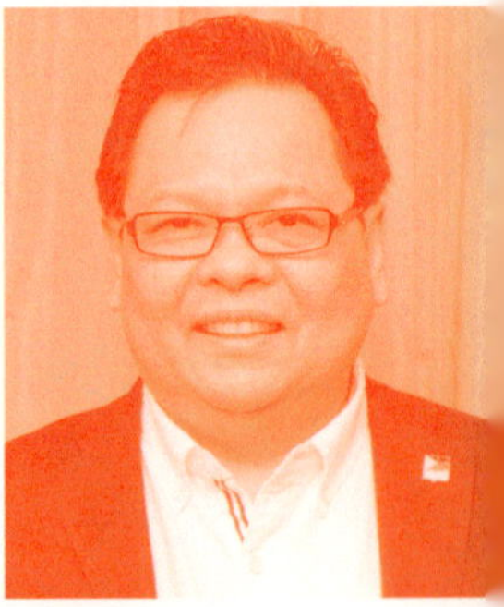

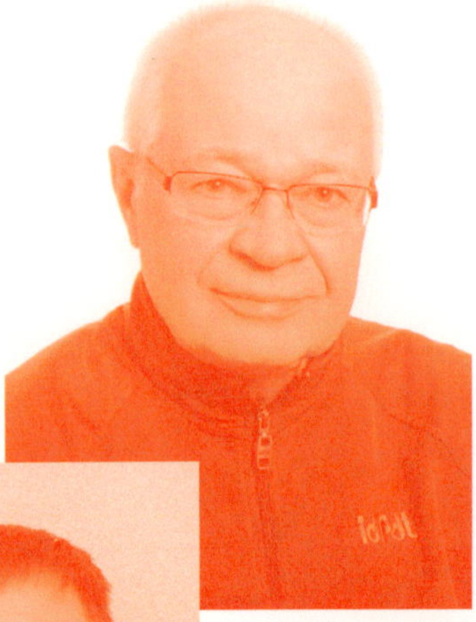

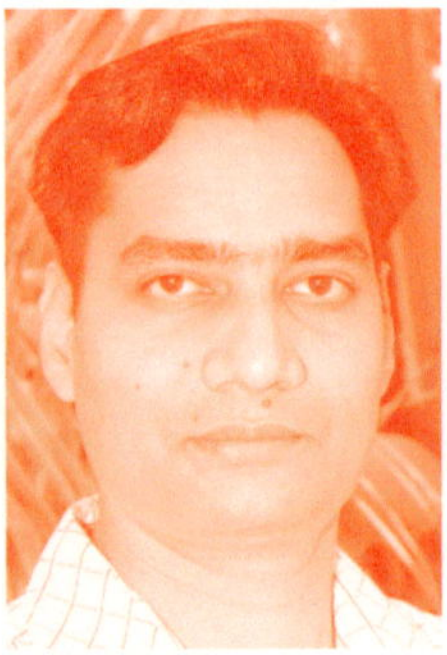

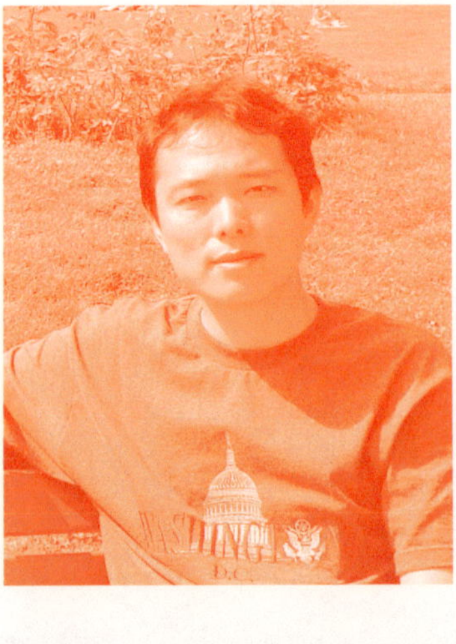

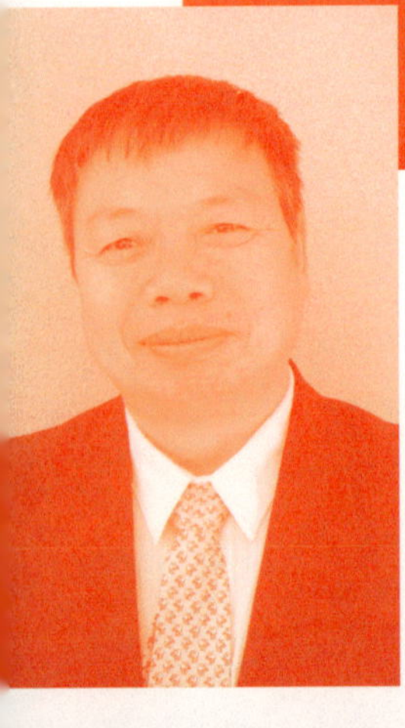

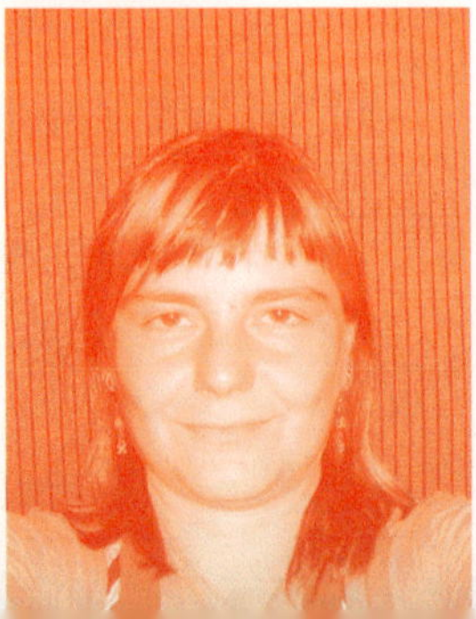

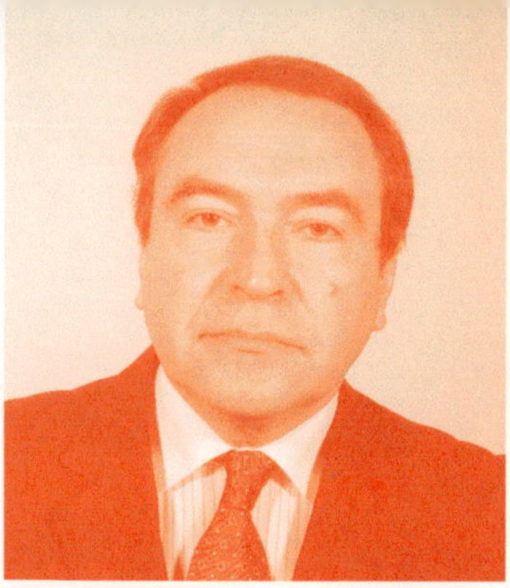
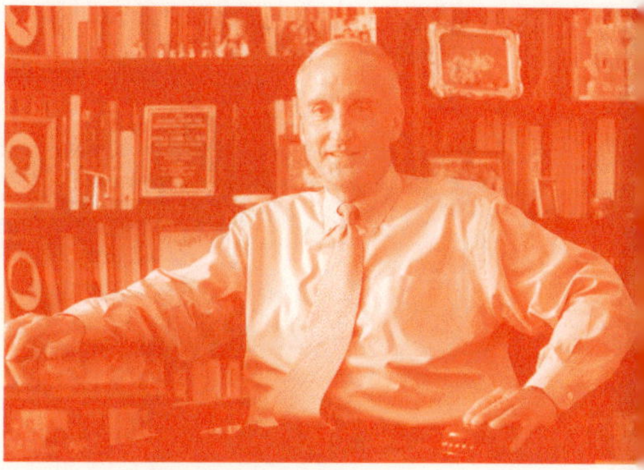
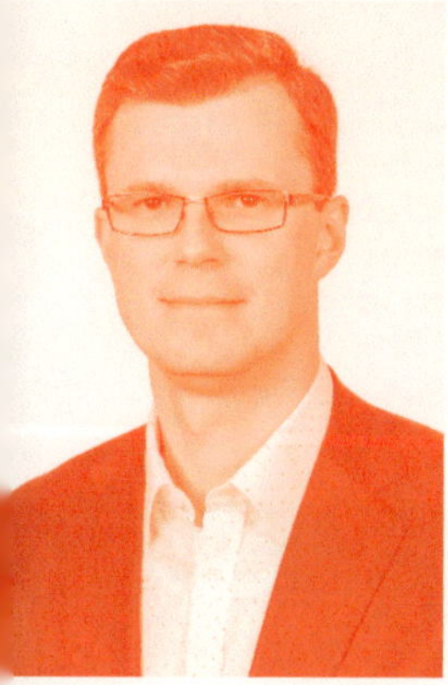
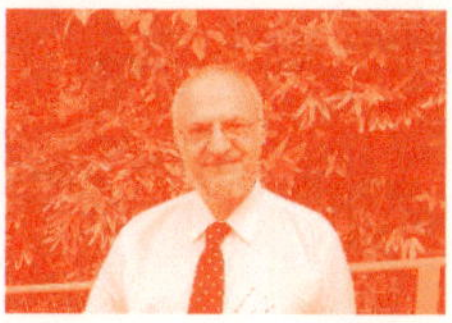
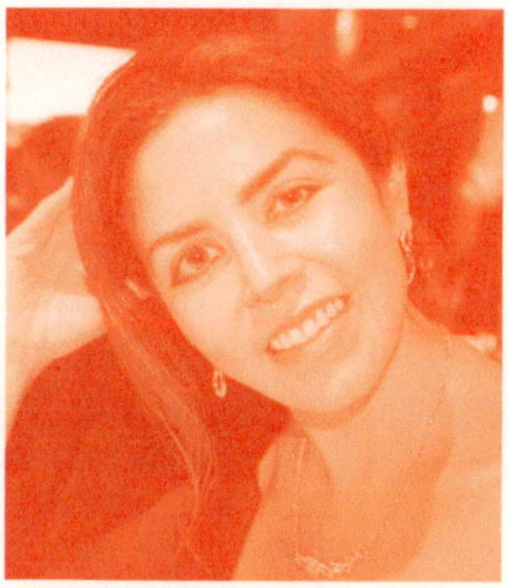

Supporting open minds since 2005

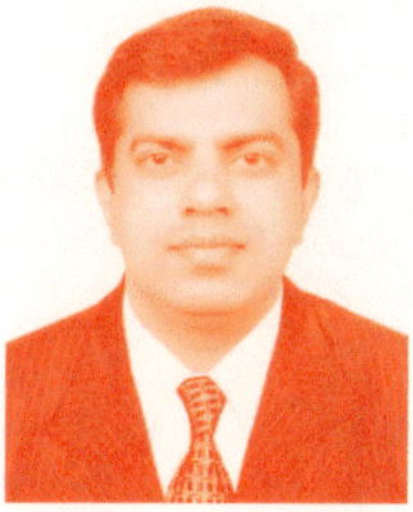
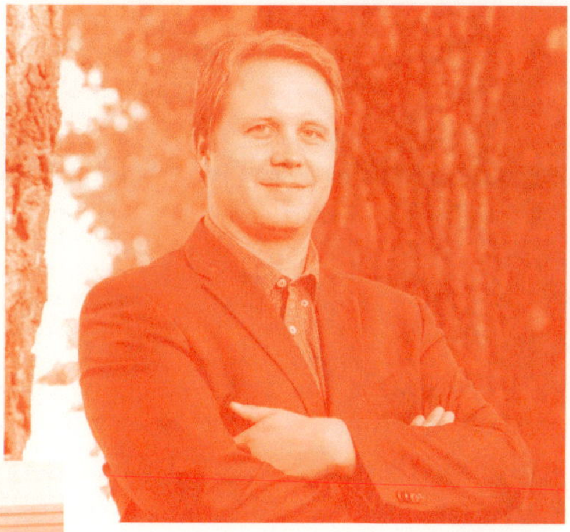
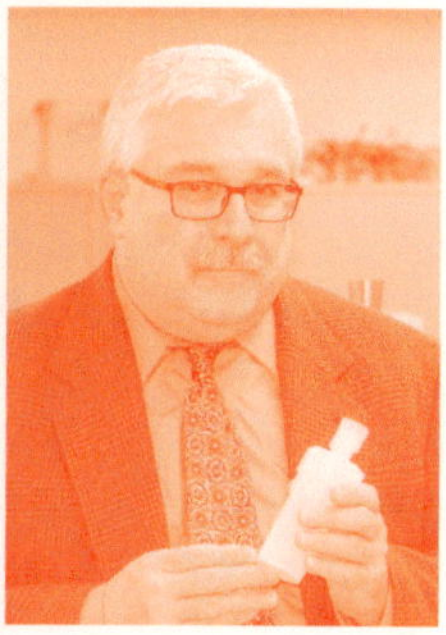
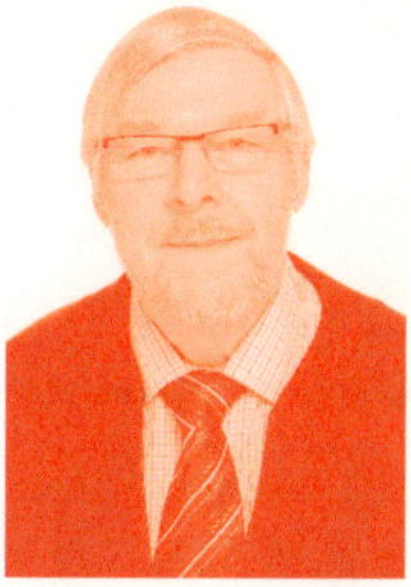
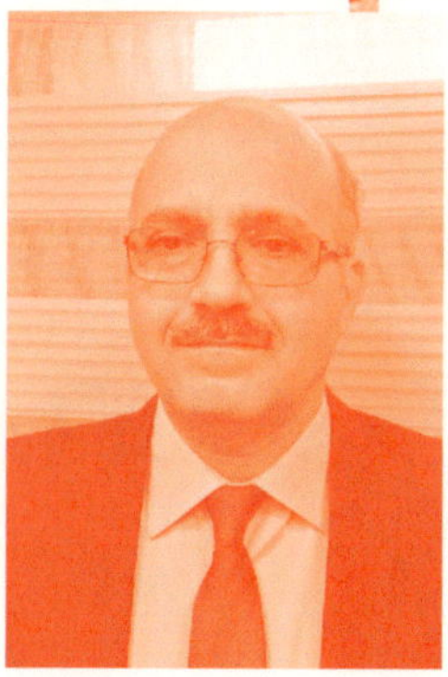
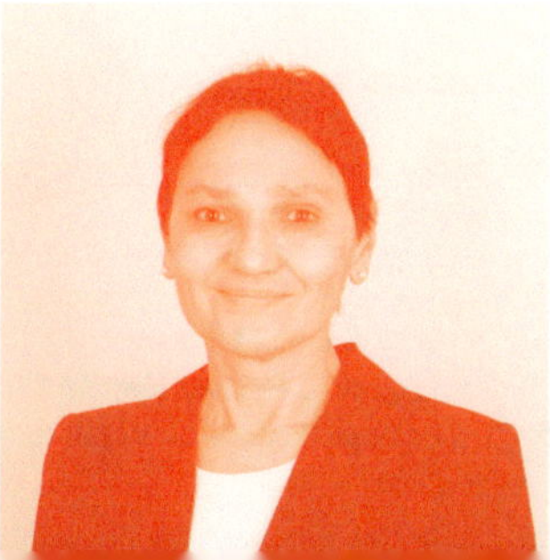
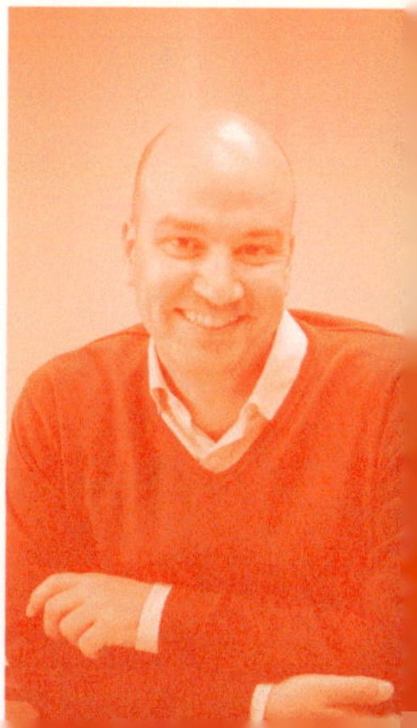

Endometriosis - Recent Advances, New Perspectives and Treatments
http://dx.doi.org/10.5772/intechopen.95742
Edited by Giovana Ap. Gonçalves

Contributors
Manuela Cristina Russu, Sushil Kumar Giri, Bhagyalaxmi Nayak, Paul-Andrei Ştefan, Roxana-Adelina Adelina Lupean, Dietmar Tamandl, David A. Trundell, Alice Ioana Albu, Dragoş Albu, Ewa J. Kleczyk, Tarachand Yadav, Stalin Amitharaj, Panagiotis Tsikouras, Fotini Gaitatzi, Stefani Filiou, Spyridon Michalopoulos, Aggeliki Gerede, Tsalikidis Christos, Stefanos Zervoudis, Anastasia Bothou, Xanthi Vatsidou, Anna Chalkidou, Georgios Dragoutsos, Ioannis Tsirkas, Konstantinos Nikolettos, Alexios Alexiou, Irine Babageorgaka, Natalia Sachnova, Theopi Nalbanti, Panagiotis Simeonidis, Nektaria Kritsotaki, Panagiotis Peitsidis, Nikolaos Nikolettos, Vasileios Souftas, Sebaidin Perende, Anastasios Vasilopoulos, Chrysovalantis Stylianou, Nikolaos Panagiotopoulos, Giovana Gonçalves, Ana Paula Girol

First published in London, United Kingdom, 2022 by IntechOpen
IntechOpen is the global imprint of INTECHOPEN LIMITED, registered in England and Wales, registration number: 11086078, 5 Princes Gate Court, London, SW7 2QJ, United Kingdom
Printed in Croatia

British Library Cataloguing-in-Publication Data
A catalogue record for this book is available from the British Library

Additional hard and PDF copies can be obtained from orders@intechopen.com

Endometriosis - Recent Advances, New Perspectives and Treatments
Edited by Giovana Ap. Gonçalves
p. cm.
Print ISBN 978-1-83969-920-7
Online ISBN 978-1-83969-921-4
eBook (PDF) ISBN 978-1-83969-922-1

For EU product safety concerns:
IN TECH d.o.o., Prolaz Marije Krucifikse Kozulić 3, 51000 Rijeka, Croatia, info@intechopen.com or visit our website at intechopen.com.

Meet the editor

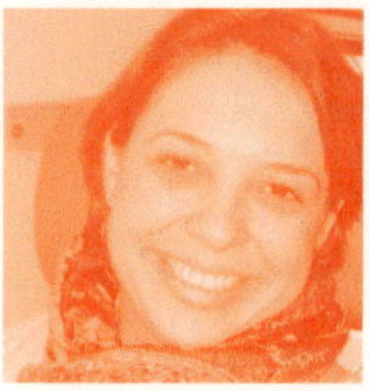

Dr. Giovana Aparecida Gonçalves is a Professor of Medicine and Nursing, at Padre Albino University Center (UNIFIPA), Brazil, and collaborating professor in the Department of Gynecology, Federal University of São Paulo State (UNIFESP), Brazil. Dr. Giovana obtained a Ph.D. in Sciences from the Heart Institute, Medical School, University of São Paulo State (USP), Brazil, in 2008; a postdoctoral degree from the Department of Gynecology, UNIFESP, in 2014; and a postdoctoral degree from Laboratory of Angiogenesis and Neurovascular Link, Vesalius Research Center–KU Leuven, Belgium, in 2015. Dr. Gonçalves develops projects in gene therapy and cell therapy with a focus on angiogenesis.

Contents

Preface

My interest in the study of endometriosis arose during my post-doc at the Department of Gynecology, Escola Paulista de Medicina, Universidade Federal de Sao Paulo (EPM-UNIFESP), Brazil, under the guidance of the late and inspiring Dr. Manoel João Batista Castello Girão (in memory) in 2008 and led me to study disease progression and cell cycle control strategies at the molecular level.

Endometriosis is not just a medical problem. Some recent research shows that there is a high chance that women surgically diagnosed with endometriosis will leave the workforce and have problems with fertility. Endometriosis is estimated to cost the world economy $9.7 billion a year. Most of these costs come from lost productivity at work. Focusing on work can be difficult due to unpredictable symptoms as well as side effects from using strong pain relievers. Women seeking a diagnosis of endometriosis through surgery need time to recover and may have more surgeries in the future.

This book presents a comprehensive overview of endometriosis, including information on molecular diagnostics and imaging methods for early detection as well as new, less-invasive treatments that preserve women's fertility.

Giovana Ap. Gonçalves
Associate Professor,
Department of Medicine – Father Albino Universitary Center - UNIFIPA,
Catanduva, Brasil

Chapter 1

Introductory Chapter: Endometriosis - Recent Advances, New Perspectives and Treatments

Giovana Ap. Gonçalves and Ana Paula Girol

1. Introduction

Endometriosis is a chronic gynecological disorder defined as the presence of endometrial tissue in extrauterine sites. Normally, functional endometrial tissue is present outside the uterine cavity and results in symptoms that include pelvic pain, dysmenorrhea, and dyspareunia. Patients with endometriosis often experience infertility and are at an increased risk of epithelial ovarian cancer. Endometriosis can be classified into three subtypes: lesions in the pelvic peritoneum; ovarian endometriosis which may occur as superficial lesions on the surface of the ovary or as cysts lined with endometrioid epithelium (endometrioma); and deeply infiltrating lesions of the rectovaginal septum [1, 2]. Despite the prevalence of endometriosis and its significant impact on women's lives, there are relatively few in vitro and in vivo models available for studying the biology and pathophysiology of this complex disease, as well as for use in the preclinical development of new therapies [3, 4].

The most accepted theory describes that viable endometrial cells, expelled by the fallopian tubes, are able to survive in the peritoneal environment by binding to its membrane [5]. However, approximately 90% of women of reproductive age with leaky fallopian tubes experience retrograde menstruation, while the prevalence of endometriosis is estimated at 6–10% [6–9]. To discover the mechanisms and propose therapeutic approaches to endometriosis, various in vitro and in vivo models of the disease are frequently proposed [9–11]. The study of endometriosis mechanisms is complex and the research results obtained may vary among different researchers who apply various methods of material collection, inclusion criteria, and genetic profiles of the sample population [12]. Furthermore, the use of primary cells in endometriosis research is highly recommended as it is a multifactorial and heterogeneous disease that varies widely among patients [5, 13–20].

In recent years, advances in neuroendocrinology, endocrinology, tumorigenesis, neurogenesis, and genomics are transforming current approaches to treating endometriosis. In this regard, GnRH antagonists, SPRM/SERM, aromatase inhibitors, immunomodulators, and antiangiogenic drugs appear as emerging and promising medical treatments for endometriosis. More studies are needed to promote personalized medication for patients with endometriosis.

One of the approaches of interest to the treatment of endometriosis is phytotherapy. The use of medicinal plants individually or in association, in the form of decoctions, extracts, and purified bioactive compounds is a common practice in several countries [21–26]. Medicinal plants exhibit many properties, including anti-inflammatory, anti-angiogenic, anti-proliferative, proapoptotic, immunomodulatory, and estrogen modulating activities which can be explored for the treatment of endometriosis or as a complementary therapy to overcome endometriosis-related symptoms [26–28]. Herbal medicines can be cheaper, easily accessible and well accepted by the population [21, 27, 28] in addition to valuing the national flora and traditions of different peoples.

Chinese herbal medicine as Xuefu Zhuyu decoction (XZD), Xiaochaihu decoction (XCHD), Qu Yi Kang (QYK), Yi Wei Ning (YWN), Yi Wei San (YWS), and Huoxue Xiaoyi decoction (HXD), which are composed of a mixture of different medicinal herbs, are widely used to relieve dysmenorrhea, reduce ectopic lesions and aid in the maintenance of fertility [21]. In general, these drugs inhibit adhesion, aggregation, and angiogenesis, reduce serum estradiol levels and inflammatory chemical mediators [21].

Angelica sinensis (Danggui), *Curcuma longa* (Jianghuang), *Pueraria lobata* (Gegen), *Salvia miltiorrhiza* (Danshen), *Paeonia lactiflora* Pall (Chishao) are some of the herbs commonly used in Chinese medicine prescriptions for dysmenorrhea and irregular menstruation due to endometriosis and which have antiangiogenic effects, including the regulation of the vascular endothelial growth factor (VEGF) [27, 29].

Additionally, bioactive compounds isolated from plants, including Epigallocatechin Gallate (catechin, *Camelia sinensis*, green and black teas), Curcumin (hydrophobic polyphenol, *Curcuma longa*), Puerarin (isoflavone from roots of *Pueraria spp*), Ginsenoside Rg3 (kind of steroid glycosides, and triterpene saponins, genus *Panax*), Resveratrol (a natural phytoalexin, mainly extracted from grapes), Genistein (isoflavone isolated from soy); Xanthohumol (*Humulus lupulus*), Naringenin (flavanones group, found in citrus and grapes) have been evaluated for the treatment of endometriosis in *in vivo* and *in vitro* models, as well as clinical trials [21, 27–31]. The actions of these bioactive compounds involve reducing the expression of VEGF, matrix metalloproteinases (MMP2 and MMP9), intercellular adhesion molecule 1 (ICAM-1) and cytokines as tumor necrosis factor-alpha (TNF-α), interleukins (IL-6 and IL-8) and monocyte chemoattractant protein 1(MCP-1) [21, 26–30].

Using bioinformatics and data mining various combinations and mechanisms of action of Chinese herbal medicines were analyzed to establish interactions with multiple targets. These studies showed that, among other findings, Chinese herbal medicines could regulate various signaling pathways including VEGF, nuclear factor kappa B (NF-κB), mitogen-activated protein kinase (MAPK), phosphatidylinositol 3-kinase (PI3K)/protein kinase B (AKT), and hypoxia-inducible factor 1 (HIF-1) [32].

In the search for new therapeutic strategies, experimental models are useful tools for understanding the effects, mechanisms of action, and safety in the use of medicinal herbs in endometriosis. However, they do not replace clinical trials, even less explored. In view of the vast literature and in order not to be exhaustive, below, only some of the investigations on herbal medicines and bioactive compounds are presented, as an example of the possibilities of treatments for endometriosis.

Regarding the traditional Chinese medicine, low and high doses of Gui Xiong Xiaoyi Wan (GXXYW), a formula that contains a combination of 14 types of plants, orally given for 28 days to rats surgically-induced endometriosis, were able to reduce the volume of the lesion, inhibit cell proliferation, induce apoptosis of endometriotic cells, as well to regulate the cell-mediated immune response by increasing the CD4:CD8 lymphocytes ratio [33]. The reduced size of the endometriotic implants was also observed for Hua Yu Xiao Zheng (HYXZ) decoction, a mixture of 13 plants, which were used in a rat endometriosis model, administered by oral gavage at three different doses. HYXZ effects are associated with decreased protein and mRNA levels of VEGF and angiopoietin 2 (Ang-2) [34].

Through nuclear magnetic resonance spectroscopy-based metabolomics, the Gui-Zhi-Fu-Ling-Capsules (GZFLC), a classic Chinese medicinal formula composed of five herbs was studied in experimental endometriosis. This study pointed out that GZFLC regulates endometriosis by modulating metabolites changes of glycolysis or gluconeogenesis and then the expression of transforming growth factor-beta 1 (TGF-β1), glucose transporter-4 (GLUT-4), and VEGF [35]. Network pharmacology and mRNA transcriptome analysis were performed to study ELeng Capsule (ELC), another Chinese medicine formula that has been used for the treatment of endometriosis [36]. Based on network pharmacology, the ELC mechanisms involve neuroactive ligand-receptor interaction, toll-like receptor, VEGF and MAPK signaling pathways related to apoptosis, angiogenesis inhibition, and immune regulation. Moreover, based on RNA-sequence analysis, ELC effects were related to regulation of cytoskeleton, epithelial-mesenchymal transition, and focal adhesion [36].

In a clinical trial, a formulation containing five Chinese medicinal plants was orally taken by post-operative women with stage III-IV endometriosis after conservative surgery, at one dosage a day for 12 consecutive weeks, and compared with anterior abdominal subcutaneous injection with goserelin acetate sustained-release depot, at the dosage of 3.6 mg once every 28 days also for 12 weeks [37]. Serum levels of cancer antigen 125 (CA-125) and IL-18 were decreased by both treatments, but between them, CA-125 levels were reduced in the herbal treated women, pointing out the effects of Chinese medicinal plants in preventing the recurrence of stage III-IV endometriosis after conservative surgery [37].

Besides Chinese medicine, several other plant extracts and bioactive compounds have been explored in preclinical investigations. *Salvia miltiorrhiza* extracts were studied in a rat endometriosis model with interesting effects as decreased serum levels of CA-125 while in peritoneal fluids IL-18 and TNF-α were reduced and IL-13, an anti-inflammatory cytokine, was increased [38]. Extracts and extracts subfractions of *Anthemis austriaca* flowers, a Turkey native plant, were applied to treat rats after surgically-induced endometriosis. Adhesion scores, endometriotic implant volumes, TNF-a, VEGF, and IL-6 levels decreased after treatments with ethyl acetate and methanol extracts and methanol subfractions. These actions may be related to flavonoids and sterols [31].

The root aqueous extract of *Entada Africana* (EA), administered at three different doses and periods, was also evaluated in an experimental model of endometriosis and indicated EA as a potential treatment of pelvic pain and female infertility. EA decreased endometrial implant volume, dysmenorrhea, prevented the progress of endometriosis by increasing the activity of catalase in endometrial implants as well as promoted ovarian follicle growth, and prevented anovulation [22]. Similarly, the ethanol extract of *Persea americana* (avocado) seeds was orally administered at different doses to treat rats with endometriosis. Again, decreased endometrial implant volume was observed, in addition to reduced ectopic endometrium heigh. Moreover, serum levels of estradiol and progesterone and luteinized unruptured follicles were reduced while the number of antral follicles and corpora lutea increased, indicating the beneficial effects of the extract [24]. Furthermore, decreased endometriotic implants volume and intra-abdominal adhesions were observed by treatment with ethyl acetate and methanol extracts obtained from flowers of *Teucrium chamaedrys* L. These effects are probably associated with secondary metabolites of nonpolar and polar features in the extracts [39].

The beneficial action of *Allium sativum* (garlic) extract on reducing the symptoms of endometriosis was clinically evaluated. The patients received usual care supplemented by a garlic tablet (400 mg of dried garlic powder; 1100 μg of allicin) daily and were followed up for 3 months. Garlic tablets reduced pelvic and back pain, dysmenorrhea, and dyspareunia [25].

The molecular docking for active ingredients of *Scurrula atropurpurea* showed that among the nine studied ingredients which can interact with the complex NF-κB/inhibitor of nuclear factor-κB (IκB), Rutin showed the strongest interaction and therefore the greatest anti-inflammatory potential [23]. However, when pure Rutin and *Uncaria guianensis* aqueous extracts obtained from bark, roots, and leaves were tested, alone or in combination, in primary stromal cells isolated from patients with and without endometriosis, using two- and three-dimensional culture models, they increased pro-inflammatory cytokines, growth factors levels, and reactive oxygen species (ROS) production. The authors speculate that cell death might increase with longer treatment time. Another consideration is that stromal and epithelial cells are present in endometriosis and the study was performed only with stromal cells [40]. Differently, in surgically-induced endometriosis, Rutin treatment enhanced apoptosis, especially at higher doses, by reducing B-cell lymphoma protein 2 (Bcl-2) and increasing Bcl-2-associated X (Bax) and cleaved caspase 9. The compound was also effective in increasing antioxidants concentrations [41].

Regarding other phytochemicals, the therapeutic potential of Curcumina was evaluated in primary cultures of stromal cells derived from eutopic endometrium of endometriosis and normal endometrial stromal cells. In a dose-dependently manner and over the time course Curcumina abrogated various chemokines, cytokines, and growth factors secretion, besides decreasing phosphorylation of the inhibitor of NF-κB kinase subunit α/β (IKKα/β), NF-κB, signal transducer and activator of transcription 3 (STAT3), and Jun N-terminal kinase (JNK) signaling molecules [42]. In addition, the treatment of rats with a protoberberine-rich fraction obtained from *Chelidonium majus* L. in an endometriosis model prevented the reoccurrence of endometriosis and positively regulated the metabolism of glucose, lactate, and glutamate [43].

As described, there are a large number of herbal medicines already in use, but which need more clinical tests to better understand their effects and mechanisms of action. Additionally, many other medicinal herbs and bioactive compounds derived from them with potential application in endometriosis are under investigation and many others can still be studied. It is important to highlight that, although extremely useful, studies in experimental models need the complementation of clinical trials so that the results can be effectively understood. These researches, associated with the enormous wealth of plant-derived products, and based on traditional knowledge, may provide new therapeutic alternatives suitable for different stages of the disease and diverse populations, which encourages the continuity of studies of herbal medicines in the management of endometriosis.

Author details

Giovana Ap. Gonçalves[1]* and Ana Paula Girol[2]

1 Centro Universitário Padre Albino—UNIFIPA, São Paulo, Brazil

2 Universidade Federal de São Paulo—UNIFESP, São Paulo, Brazil

*Address all correspondence to: goncalves.giovana2@gmail.com

References

[1] Falconer H, D'Hooghe T, Fried G. Endometriosis and genetic polymorphisms. Obstetrical & Gynecological Survey. 2007;**62**(9): 616-628

[2] Ulukus M, Cakmak H, Arid A. The role of endometrium in endometriosis. The Journal of the Society for Gynecologic Investigation: JSGI. 2006;**13**(7):467-476

[3] Giudice LC et al. Genetics and genomics of endometriosis. Human reproductive and prenatal. Genetics. 2019:399-426

[4] Kao LC, Giudice LC. Articletitle endometriosis. Lancet. 2004;**364**: 1789-1799

[5] Sampson JA. Peritoneal endometriosis due to the menstrual dissemination of endometrial tissue into the peritoneal cavity. American Journal of Obstetrics & Gynecology. 1927;**14**(4):422-469

[6] Halme J et al. Retrograde menstruation in healthy women and in patients with endometriosis. Obstetrics and Gynecology. 1984;**64**(2):151-154

[7] Liu DTY, Hitchcock A. Endometriosis: Its association with retrograde menstruation, dysmenorrhoea and tubal pathology. Bjog: An International Journal of Obstetrics & Gynaecology. 1986;**93**(8):859-862

[8] Watkins RE. Uterine retrodisplacements, retrograde menstruation and endometriosis. West Journal of Surgery, Obstetrics and Gynecology. 1938;**46**:480-494

[9] Zondervan KT et al. Endometriosis. Nature Reviews Disease Primers. 2018

[10] Griffith JS, Rodgers AK, Schenken RS. In vitro models to study the pathogenesis of endometriosis. Reproductive Sciences. 2010;**17**(1):5-12

[11] Grümmer R. Models of endometriosis: In vitro and in vivo models. Endometriosis: Science and Practice. 2012:263-269

[12] Miller LM, Johnson NP. Ephect–The endometriosis phenome (and biobanking) harmonisation project– May be very helpful for clinicians and the women they are treating. F1000research, V. 6, 2017

[13] D'amora P et al. Disrupted cell cycle control in cultured endometrial cells from patients with endometriosis harboring the progesterone receptor polymorphism progins. The American Journal of Pathology. 2009;**175**(1): 215-224

[14] Gonçalves GA. Molecular basis of endometriosis: The intergration of Research and Clinical Pratice. IntechOpen. Bod-Books On Demand. 2019

[15] Gonçalves GA. P27kip1 as a key regulator of endometriosis. European Journal of Obstetrics & Gynecology and Reproductive Biology. 2018;**221**:1-4

[16] Gonçalves GA et al. P27 Kip1 overexpression regulates Vegf expression, cell proliferation and apoptosis in cell culture from eutopic endometrium of women with endometriosis. Apoptosis. 2015;**20**(3):327-335

[17] Guo SW, Groothuis PG. Is it time for a paradigm shift in drug research and development in endometriosis/ adenomyosis? Human Reproduction Update. 2018;**24**(5):577-598

[18] Jibrim RLM et al. Expression of the Tfdp1 gene in the endometrium of women with deep infiltrating

endometriosis. Gynecological Endocrinology. 2019;**35**(6):490-493

[19] Kopelman A et al. Analysis of gene expression in the endocervical epithelium of women with deep endometriosis. Reproductive Sciences. 2016;**23**(9):1269-1274

[20] Luckow Invitti A et al. Inflammatory cytokine profile of co-cultivated primary cells from the endometrium of women with and without endometriosis. Molecular Medicine Reports. 2018;**18**(2):1287-1296

[21] Kong S, Zhang Y-H, Liu C-F, Tsui I, Guo Y, Ai B-B, et al. The complementary and alternative medicine for endometriosis: A review of utilization and mechanism. Evidence-Based Complementary and Alternative Medicine. 2014: Article ID: 146383, 16 p

[22] Mvondo MA, Essono SM, Tatsinkou FDB, Ateba SB, Njamen D. The root aqueous extract of Entada Africana Guill. Et Perr. (Mimosaceae) inhibits implant growth, alleviates dysmenorrhea, and restores ovarian dynamic in a rat model of endometriosis. Evidence-Based Complementary and Alternative Medicine. 2017: Article ID: 8563909, 15 p. DOI: 10.1155/2017/8563909

[23] Yuniwati C, Ramli N, Purwita E, Yusnaini Y, Nurdahliana N, Miko A, et al. Molecular docking for active compounds of scurrula atropurpurea as anti-inflammatory candidate in endometriosis. Acta Informatica Medica. 2018;**26**(4):254-257

[24] Essono SM, Mvondo MA, Ngadjui E, Nguimatio FXK, Watcho P. The ethanol extract of avocado (*Persea Americana* Mill. (Lauraceae)) seeds successfully induces implant regression and restores ovarian dynamic in a rat model of endometriosis. Evidence-Based Complementary and Alternative Medicine Volume. 2020: Article ID: 8521831, 10 p. DOI: 10.1155/2020/8521831

[25] Amirsalari S, Moghadam ZB, Taghizadeh Z, Abadi MNJ, Irani PS, Goodarzi S, et al. The effect of garlic tablets on the endometriosis-related pains: A Randomized Placebo-Controlled Clinical Trial. Evidence-Based Complementary and Alternative Medicine. 2021: Article ID: 5547058, 8 p. DOI: 10.1155/2021/5547058

[26] Ilhan M, Dereli FTG, Akkol EK. Novel drug targets with traditional herbal medicines for overcoming endometriosis. Current Drug Delivery. 2019;**16**:386-399

[27] Balan A, Moga MA, Dima L, Dinu CG, Martinescu CC, Panait DE, et al. An overview on the conservative management of endometriosis from a naturopathic perspective: Phytochemicals and medicinal plants. Plants. 2021;**10**:587

[28] Gołabek A, Kowalska K, Olejnik A. Polyphenols as a diet therapy concept for endometriosis. Current opinion and future perspectives. Nutrients. 2021;**13**:1347

[29] Zheng W, Cao L, Xu Z, Ma Y, Liang X. Anti-angiogenic alternative and complementary medicines for the treatment of endometriosis: A review of potential molecular mechanisms. Evidence-Based Complementary and Alternative Medicine. 2018: Article ID: 4128984, 28 p

[30] Bartiromo L, Schimberni M, Villanacci R, Ottolina J, Dolci C, Salmeri N, et al. Endometriosis and phytoestrogens: Friends or foes? A Systematic Review Nutrients. 2021;**13**:2532

[31] Ilhan M, Ali Z, Khan IA, Tastan H, Akkol EK. Promising activity of anthemis Austriaca Jacq. on the endometriosis rat model and isolation

of its active constituents. Saudi Pharmaceutical Journal. 2019;**27**:889-899

[32] Zheng W, Wu J, Gu J, Weng H, Wang J, Wang T, et al. Modular characteristics and mechanism of action of herbs for endometriosis treatment in Chinese medicine: A data mining and network pharmacology–based identification. Frontiers in Pharmacology. 2020;**11**:147. DOI: 10.3389/Fphar.2020.00147

[33] Jin Z, Wang L, Zhu Z. Effect of Guixiong Xiaoyi Wan in treatment of endometriosis on rats. Evidence-Based Complementary And Alternative Medicine. 2015: Article ID: 208514, 8 p. DOI: 10.1155/2015/208514

[34] Chen Z-Z, Gong X. Effect of Hua Yu Xiao Zheng Decoction on the expression levels of vascular endothelial growth factor and Angiopoietin-2 in rats with endometriosis. Experimental and Therapeutic Medicine. 2017;**14**: 5743-5750

[35] Zhou J, Ding Z-M, Hardiman PJ. Understanding the role of Gui-Zhi-Fu-Ling-Capsules (Chinese Medicine) for treatment of endometriosis in the rat model: Using NMR based metabolomics. Evidence-Based Complementary and Alternative Medicine. 2018: Article ID: 9864963, 9 p. DOI: 10.1155/2018/9864963

[36] Zheng W, Wang J, Wu J, Wang T, Huang Y, Liang X, et al. Exploration of the modulatory property mechanism of eleng capsule in the treatment of endometriosis using transcriptomics combined with systems network pharmacology. Frontiers in Pharmacology. 2021;**12**:674874. DOI: 10.3389/Fphar.2021.674874

[37] Weng Q, Ding Z-M, Lv X-L, Yang D-X, Song Y-Z, Wang F-F, et al. Chinese medicinal plants for advanced endometriosis after conservative surgery: A prospective, multi-center and controlled trial. International Journal of Clinical and Experimental Medicine. 2015;**8**(7):11307-11311

[38] Zhou Z-H, Weng Q, Zhou J-H, Zhou J. Extracts of salvia miltiorrhiza bunge on the cytokines of rat endometriosis models. African Journal of Tradititional, Complementary and Alternative Medicine. 2012;**9**(3):303-314. DOI: 10.4314/ajtcam.v9i3.2303

[39] Özel Ş, Süntar İ, Gökay NE, Türkmenoğlu TT, Demırel MA. The effectiveness of *Teucrium chamaedrys* L. extracts on endometriotic implant regression in rat endometriosis model veterinary. Research Forum. 2020;**11**(4): 305-309. DOI: 10.30466/Vrf.2019.105229.2500

[40] Hernandes C, De Oliveira RN, Santos AHDS, Malvezzi H, De Azevedo BC, Gueuvoghlanian-Silva BY, et al. The effect of rutin and extracts of Uncaria Guianensis (Aubl.) J. F. Gmeland on primary endometriotic cells: A 2D and 3D study. Molecules. 2020;**25**:1325. DOI: 10.3390/Molecules.25061325

[41] Talebi H, Farahpour MR, Hamishehkar H. The efectiveness of rutin for prevention of surgical induced endometriosis development in a rat model. Scientifc Reports. 2021;**11**:7180

[42] Chowdhury I, Banerjee S, Driss A, Xu W, Mehrabi S, Nezhat C, et al. Curcumin attenuates proangiogenic and proinflammatory factors in human eutopic endometrial stromal cells through the NF-Kb signaling pathway. Journal of Cell Physiology. 2019;**234**: 6298-6312

[43] Warowicka A, Qasem B, Dera-Szymanowska A, Wołu M, Florczak P, Horst N, et al. Effect of protoberberine-rich fraction of *Chelidonium majus* L. on endometriosis regression. Pharmaceutics. 2021;**13**:931

Chapter 2

Endometriosis and Cancer

Sushil Kumar Giri and Bhagyalaxmi Nayak

Abstract

Endometriosis is a chronic debilitating inflammatory disease of women, with the growth of ectopic endometrium in extrauterine sites like rectovaginal septum, peritoneal surfaces, or ovaries, etc. Though endometriosis is not regarded as a malignant disorder, it does have some features common to malignant disease. They are; local and distant metastasis, invasion and destruction to adjacent structures, unrestricted growth, development of new blood vessels. The association between endometriosis and ovarian, endometrial, and cervical cancers and between endometriosis and extra-ovarian malignancies has been reported in different kinds of literature. Clear cell and endometrioid ovarian carcinomas are presumed to have developed from endometriosis. Ovarian seromucinous borderline tumors, low-grade serous ovarian carcinomas, adenosarcoma, and endometrial stromal sarcomas may also arise from endometriosis. However, it is not very clear whether endometriosis has undergone malignant transformation or simply is found co-existent with cancer. Endometriosis itself may increase a woman's risk of developing non-Hodgkin's lymphoma, malignant melanoma, and breast cancer.

Keywords: endometriosis, common genetic instability, cancer

1. Introduction

Endometriosis is a chronic debilitating inflammatory disease of women, with the growth of ectopic endometrium in extrauterine sites like uterosacral ligaments, pelvic peritoneum, rectovaginal septum, other peritoneal surfaces, ovaries, etc. It is an extremely heterogeneous clinical entity as regards etiopathogenesis, clinical features, and treatment. The genetic basis of this disease has been quite clear and endometriosis running in families has been quite established. The exact etiopathogenesis and treatment option of the disease is still evolving. Though endometriosis is not regarded as a malignant disorder, it does have some features akin to malignant disease. They are local and distant metastasis, invasion and destruction of adjacent structures, unrestricted growth, resistance to apoptosis, development of new blood vessels etc [1]. With the increasing availability of new gene sequencing methods, the genetic profiling of endometriosis has given way to new findings that endometriosis and certain cancers share the same aberrant genetic sequences.

Sampson et al. in 1925 postulated a histological link between endometriosis and cancer and proposed the three criteria for the diagnosis of endometriosis-associated ovarian cancer (EAOC). They were (1) evidence of endometriosis close to the tumor, (2) exclusion of invasion from other sources, (3) presence of tissue resembling endometrial stroma surrounding characteristic epithelial glands [2]. Scott et al. in 1953 revised the criteria and added the fourth criterion, i.e., histological proof of transition from benign changes in endometriosis to malignant changes [3].

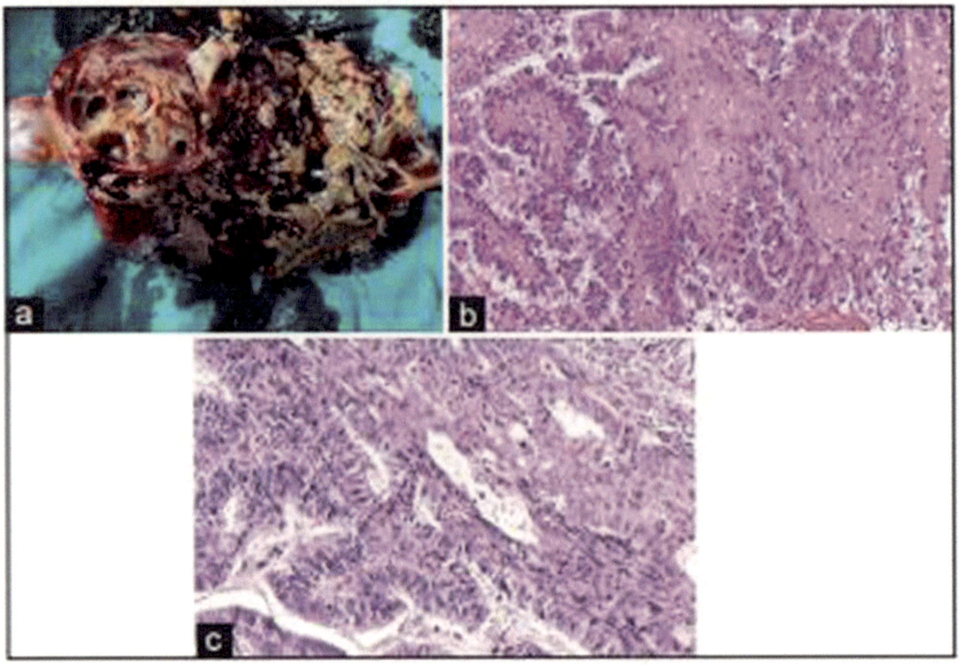

Figure 1.
(a) Cut section of an ovarian mass showing chocolate material with solid components, (b) clear cell carcinoma ovary associated with endometriosis, (c) endometrioid adenocarcinoma in the vicinity of endometriosis.

All four criteria are continued in practice to diagnose endometriosis-associated malignancy (EAM) (**Figure 1**).

Endometriosis is associated with genetic instability and several genetic alterations. Loss of heterozygosity (LOH) at 10q23, PTEN, ARID1A, and p53 mutations have been found in both endometriosis and EAM [4]. It is presumed that EAM arises from atypical endometriosis, which is an intermediate lesion between endometriosis and cancer. About 80% of EAM is found in the ovary and the rest are localized in the abdominal wall, pleura, intestine, rectovaginal septum etc [5].

Considering the above facts, obvious controversies ensue as to the role of endometriosis as the cause of malignant transformation or a mere association with cancers.

2. The mechanism for malignant transformation of endometriosis

The exact mechanisms of malignant transformation of endometriosis are not fully established. It is proposed that chronic inflammation and immune dysregulation are the main factors related to the malignant transformation of endometriosis due to most probably iron-triggered oxidative stress leading to genetic alteration [6]. It is reported that endometriotic cysts have more concentration of iron than non-endometrioid counterparts, because of periodic hemorrhage into the cyst with the accumulation of free iron. Moreover, genomic alteration also is a resultant of hyperoestrogenic state associated with endometriosis, leading to inactivation of tumor suppressor genes like p53, PTEN, ARID 1A, and activation of KRAS and p13 oncogenic pathways, thus favoring the development of hormone-dependent malignant diseases like Type-I epithelial ovarian cancer and breast cancers [7]. Some authors have also established an association of endometriosis with ovarian cancer,

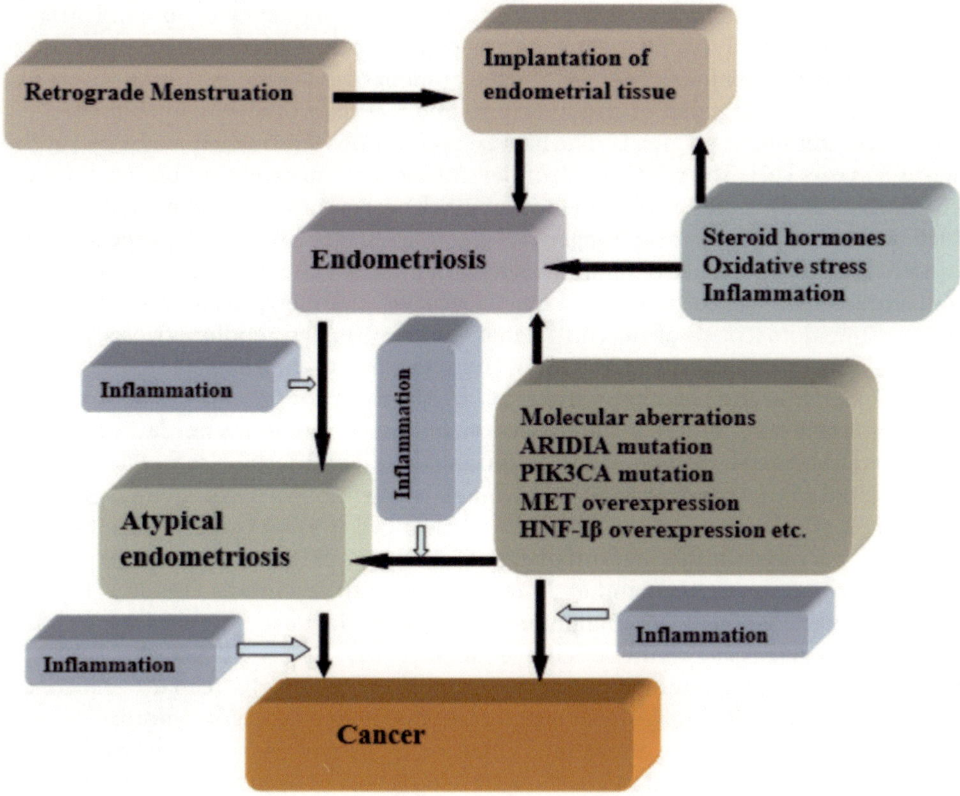

Figure 2.
Probable pathway for transformation of endometriosis to cancer.

breast cancer (BC), cutaneous melanoma, and non-Hodgkin's lymphoma [1, 8]. It is presumed that endometriosis-associated, and endometriosis independent neoplasms may develop from different molecular pathways with distinct genetic alteration with significant clinical and prognostic implications. The estrogen-dependent pathogenesis of ovarian endometrioid carcinomas associated with endometriosis is corroborated also by the increased incidence of synchronous primary endometrial (Type I, estrogen-dependent) and ovarian, endometriosis-associated, endometrioid adenocarcinomas (**Figure 2**).

3. Endometriosis and specific cancers

3.1 Endometriosis and ovarian cancer

In a recently completed large cohort study "The ENOCA population-based cohort study" analyzing 2043 women of ovarian cancer in the endometriosis cohort and 471 women with ovarian cancer in the nevus cohort, the authors observed an increased incidence of endometrioid and clear-cell ovarian cancer in women with histologically proven endometriosis and the median age of ovarian cancer diagnosis was 56 years and 60 years in endometriosis and nevus cohort respectively [9]. The exact mechanism of development of EAOC is yet to be understood. However, the presence of some factors is implicated in a higher risk of the development of EAOC. In a recent study, it was observed that increasing age, postmenopausal status, high level of CA-125, ovarian endometrioma >8 cm size, long-standing endometriosis of >5 years duration was found to have a higher risk of coexistent malignancy in both univariate and multivariate analysis. Longer use of oral contraceptive pills does have a protective effect. A significantly increased risk of development of ovarian cancer was observed after 1–4 years of diagnosis of endometriosis and 5–9 years of follow-up, but not ≥10 years after initial diagnosis. The highest risk was observed when diagnosed at the age of 50 years [10]. The relative risk of developing ovarian cancer is about 4.2 times higher than the general population in women with long-standing endometriosis and such women are 10–20 years younger [11]. To establish the EAOC, it is proposed that, in addition to the presence of ovarian cancer, there should have at least one of the following criteria: (1) coexistence of carcinoma and endometriosis within the same ovary; (2) endometriosis of the contralateral ovary, (3) pelvic endometriosis, or (4) histology-proven transition from benign endometriosis to cancer [12].

Endometrioid and clear cell carcinoma are the most common types of ovarian carcinoma of EAOC, whereas the endocervical type of mucinous borderline tumor, endometrial stromal sarcoma, and Mullerian adenosarcoma are less frequently encountered [5]. It was described that women with endometriosis have a 2–3 times higher risk of developing endometrioid and clear cell ovarian tumors [13]. It was observed in a recent study that out of EAOC, 32% and 28% constituted clear cell ovarian carcinoma (CCOC) and endometrioid ovarian carcinoma (EnOC) respectively. About 62% of ovarian malignancy cases were diagnosed in early-stage and overall optimal surgery could be achieved in 88% [11]. As CA-125 is raised both in endometriosis and carcinoma ovary, estimation of serum HE4 can differentiate between the two as its higher level is detected mostly in ovarian carcinoma.

The molecular genomic alteration, inflammation, hyperestrogenism, and oxidative stress, etc. in combination are thought to be involved in the transformation of endometriosis from benign to atypical (borderline) and then to EAOC [11]. Other risk factors involved are obesity and the use of unopposed estrogen. EAOC develops from atypical endometriosis with common molecular alteration such as mutations of ARID1A, PI3KCA, and loss of heterozygosity of PTEN, hepatocyte nuclear factor-1b (HNF-1b) upregulation, and mutation of CTNNB1 (catenin beta 1) [14]. However, a higher frequency of ARID1A mutations of 46–57% has been observed in CCOC in comparison to 30% in EnOC [15]. In both situations, atypical endometriosis has been identified as a direct precursor [16].

Diagnosis of malignant transformation in endometriosis or endometrioma is very challenging. Some degree of caution should be exercised in women at high risk of malignant transformation, like women with a long-standing history, endometriosis diagnosed at an early age, large endometrioma, endometriosis-associated infertility, and/or history of infertility treatment. Early detection is of paramount importance to improve the prognosis. As the EAOC presents at an early stage, optimal cytoreduction is feasible, and fertility promoting surgery is possible as the case may demand. Features of malignant transformation can be picked up by high-resolution ultrasound and by expert ultrasonologist. In a retrospective multicenter study involving 239 women of endometrioid carcinoma, the authors observed unilocular cyst with papillary projection without ascites in most instances of EAOC, whereas endometrioid carcinoma without evidence of endometriosis had a large central solid component entrapped within locules, giving the tumor a cockade-like appearance [17]. Unilateral cystic mass containing hemorrhagic fluid and mural nodule is the characteristic feature of T1 weighted images of contrast-enhanced MRI in the diagnosis of malignant transformation of endometrioma. The disappearance of shading on T2-weighted images with enlargement of endometrioma is suggestive of malignant transformation [18].

The long-standing persistence of endometriosis plays an important role in the development of EAOC. It was observed that there is an increased risk of development of both EnOC and CCOC after 10 years of diagnosis of endometriosis. Moreover, when the first diagnosis of endometriosis is at 50 years or more, there is an increased risk of serous ovarian cancer, though the increased risk of CCOC was observed in all age groups at first diagnosis of endometriosis [8].

Some authors observed that EAOCs present in the low stage and low-grade disease status with a significantly better prognosis compared with non-EAOC counterparts [19]. However, other experts had contradictory views and opined that the better outcome was due to early-stage and grade of the disease and not because of associated endometriosis [20]. Surgery followed by standard chemotherapy is the treatment of choice when deemed necessary, though the response to chemotherapy is not so encouraging. However, in a large population-based cohort study, longer survival was observed in ovarian cancer patients with histologically proven endometriosis than those without endometriosis even after adjusting stage, grade, type, age at diagnosis, treatment protocol, and residual tumor after surgery [9]. Given the poor response to standard chemotherapy and as mutation of ARID1A, PI3K/AKT/mTOR, MET, and HNF-1β pathways are frequently activated, targeted inhibitors for these pathways can be considered as a future in the treatment strategy for EAOC, especially OCCC [21].

It will not be out of the place to mention that most women with endometriosis will not develop carcinoma of the ovary. Though evidence from several studies demonstrates increased risk, the lifetime risk of developing ovarian cancer is still low in women with endometriosis and is not different from women without endometriosis. The clinician and the woman need to be aware of the risk, but need not be worried about the cancer risk [22].

3.1.1 Prevention strategies for EAOC

As of now, there is no availability of any specific biological markers to stratify which endometriosis case will develop into a malignant one. A recently published report suggests that ovarian endometriosis is prone to develop into ovarian cancer, while there is no association between peritoneal or deep endometriosis and ovarian cancer [23]. As mutations in ARID1A, PTEN, PIK3CA, and KRAS are associated both in endometriosis and ovarian cancer of the same patient, detection of these and other mutations may predict future development of EAOC.

The application of sensitive and specific molecular biomarkers needs to be explored to identify endometriosis with oncogenic potential. Employing the study of circulating tumor DNA (ctDNA) can play a major role in detecting cancer precursor lesions present in some endometriosis [24]. Few interventions can reduce the risk of ovarian cancer in general and EAOC in particular. It is evident that 5 years of use of oral contraceptive pills results in a 20–30% reduction of EnOC and CCC [25]. Tubal ligation shows almost 50% risk reduction of EnOC and CCC [26]. Risk-reducing salpingo-oophorectomy may be considered in endometriosis to prevent EAOC as well as symptom relief. Unilateral oophorectomy with complete resection of all visible endometriotic lesions has been observed to have a protective effect in the development of ovarian cancer [27]. As the risk of development of ovarian cancer is more when endometriosis is detected in women aged ≥50 years, complete surgical resection is of paramount importance in older women diagnosed with endometriosis [28].

3.2 Endometriosis and endometrial carcinoma

Pathogenesis of both endometriosis and endometrial carcinoma is not well defined and thought to be multifactorial with an uncertain underlying molecular mechanism. However, mutation of the gene as observed in EAOC has been identified to be associated with endometrioid endometrial carcinoma [29]. Both estrogen stimulation and chronic inflammation have been attributed as causative factors of the two disorders. The endometrioid histopathology of co-existent ovarian and endometrial carcinoma (synchronous) with evidence of ovarian endometriosis in 30% of cases points towards the association of endometriosis and endometrial cancer [30]. J.B. Mogensen, et al. [7] observed a statistically significant increased risk of development of mostly Type-I endometrial carcinoma after 10 years of initial diagnosis of endometriosis [7]. They detected a 40% increased risk of endometrial carcinoma as opposed to other studies showing no association [31]. H.C. Yu HC.et al. had the same observation of the increased association of endometriosis and endometrial cancer [32]. A. Dahiya et al. detected 104 (13%) cases of different malignancies from 800 patients of histologically proven endometriosis. Out of which 33 cases had endometrial carcinoma with endometrioid histology in 87.8% of cases and 81.8% were in stage I [10]. In a population-based retrospective cohort study of 129,862 women with histologically proven endometriosis/adenomyosis, M. Hermens et al. observed an increased incidence of endometrial cancer. They suggested evaluating endometrium before hysterectomy for endometriosis to exclude endometrial carcinoma so that inappropriate surgery can be avoided [33].

3.3 Endometriosis and breast cancer

Data are inconsistent to establish a relationship between endometriosis and breast cancer [34]. Both are associated with a high oestrogenic environment. Farland et al. in their prospective cohort study did not find an increased risk of ER & PR+ve, or ER & PR−ve breast cancer in women with laparoscopically proved endometriosis in a follow-up period of 24 years. Rather they observed an increased risk of ER+ve and PR−ve breast cancers in women with endometriosis [35].

3.4 Endometriosis and cervical cancer

Saavalainen et al. found a strongly decreased risk of squamous cell carcinoma of the cervix in women diagnosed with peritoneal endometriosis. This can be explained that screening for cervical cancer as such can have an impact on such reduction and reduced sexual activity, because of dyspareunia, thereby reducing exposure to HPV infection [23].

3.5 Endometriosis and non-gynecological cancers

The association of endometriosis and non-gynecological cancers is not well established nor well studied. However, some association has been attributed in some studies as described below.

3.5.1 Endometriosis and colorectal cancer (CRC)

In a prospective study of 2266 women with endometriosis, with 9842 patient-years of follow-up, a marked (13-fold) increase in the incidence of CRC was observed in women with adenomyosis and extragonadal endometriosis. This is attributed to the malignant transformation of endometriotic implants over colorectal tissue, partly due to the hyperoestrogenic environment [36].

3.5.2 Non-Hodgkin's lymphoma

A study by J.E. Olson et al. reported 3.2 times increased risk of development of diffuse non-Hodgkin's lymphoma and extranodal disease in women with endometriosis as compared to those without it [37]. A similar observation was described by A. Melin et al. in their study using National Swedish Inpatient Register [38]. They linked this association to abnormal cellular and humoral immune function. As polyclonal B-cell autoimmune activation is observed in endometriosis, it is postulated to associate B cell lymphoma to B cell activation of endometriosis.

3.5.3 Endometriosis and Thyroid Cancer

In a large cohort study from the Finish Cancer registry, L. Saavalainen et al. observed an increased risk of thyroid cancer especially of papillary type in women with diagnosed endometriosis [39]. Women do have three times more risk of development of thyroid cancer than men and attribute it to female sex hormones. So hormonal abnormality, mostly estrogen disorder may be a risk factor for thyroid cancer, which is also a factor for endometriosis [40].

3.5.4 Endometriosis and brain tumor

Melin et al. in a large study demonstrated the association of endometriosis to brain tumour [41]. E.B. Claus et al. in a large study observed endometriosis as a risk factor for meningioma and attributed hormonal factors for such incidence [42].

3.5.5 Endometriosis and skin cancer

L.V. Farland et al. observed that women with endometriosis do have an increased risk of skin cancers, mostly associated with melanoma. They also found no association of endometriosis with basal cell carcinoma and squamous cell carcinoma [43]. A similar association was also observed by M. Kvaskoff et al. They attributed hormonal hypothesis and some molecular genetic alteration in both the conditions [44].

3.5.6 Endometriosis and other cancers

Saavalainen et al. observed a 40% decreased risk of oral and pharynx carcinoma. This decrease might be due to less exposure to HPV infection and complex alteration of immune response associated with HPV and endometriosis. Though not HPV-related, about ⅕th decrease in the incidence of pancreatic carcinoma was observed in women with endometriosis. The cause of this lower risk might be attributed to lifestyle modification and hormonal treatment for endometriosis [23].

4. Conclusion

The link between endometriosis and different cancers is yet to be well understood. Though evidence dates back to the early 1990s, we still need robust data to back the hypothesis. Genetic alteration and hormonal role are postulated to be factors in the development of different cancers in women with endometriosis. The exact mechanism of this complex process is yet to be established. First, we need to understand the basics of endometriosis, the physiological changes, genetic aberration associated with the disease, and morbidity issues. All women with endometriosis should be evaluated clinically and with appropriate imaging studies and be managed appropriately by specific drugs, fertility-enhancing surgery, or surgical removal of all visible lesions which may necessitate hysterectomy and bilateral oophorectomy. These women need strict follow-up even years after menopause. This will reduce the risk of future development of EAOC. More methodically robust prospective research with a large population is the need of the day to attribute the relationship of endometriosis and cancers as a cause or association. Our knowledge is growing and our understanding is evolving.

Author details

Sushil Kumar Giri* and Bhagyalaxmi Nayak
PG Department of Gynaecologic Oncology, A.H. Postgraduate Institute of Cancer, Cuttack, Odisha, India

*Address all correspondence to: drskgiri@gmail.com

References

[1] Kvaskoff M, Mu F, Terry KL, Harris HR, Poole EM, Farland L, et al. Endometriosis: A high-risk population for major chronic diseases? Human Reproduction Update. 2015;**21**:500-516

[2] Sampson JA. Endometrial carcinoma of the ovary arising in endometrial tissue in that organ. Archives of Surgery. 1925;**10**:1-7

[3] Scott RB. Malignant changes in endometriosis. Obstetrics and Gynecology. 1953;**2**:283-289

[4] Pollacco J, Sacco K, Portelli M, Schembri-Wismayer P, Calleja-Agius J. Molecular links between endometriosis and cancer. Gynecological Endocrinology. 2012;**28**:577-581

[5] Krawczyk N, Banys-Paluchowski M, Schmidt D, Ulrich U, Fehm T. Endometriosis-associated malignancy. Geburtsh Frauenheilk. 2016;**76**:176-181

[6] Vercellini P, Viganò P, Somigliana E, Fedele L. Endometriosis: Pathogenesis and treatment. Nature Reviews. Endocrinology. 2014;**10**(5):26

[7] Mogensen JB, Kjær SK, Mellemkjær L, Jensen A. Endometriosis and risks for ovarian, endometrial and breast cancers: A nationwide cohort study. Gynecologic Oncology. 2016;**143**(1):8

[8] Kokcu A. Relationship between endometriosis and cancer from a current perspective. Archives of Gynecology and Obstetrics. 2011;**284**:1473-1479

[9] Hermens M, van Altena AM, Nieboer TE, Schoot BC, van Vliet HAAM, Siebers AG, et al. Incidence of endometrioid and clear-cell ovarian cancer in histological proven endometriosis. The ENOCA population-based cohort study. American Journal of Obstetrics and Gynecology. 2020 Jul;**223**(1):107.e1-107. DOI: 10.1016/j.ajog.2020.01.041

[10] Dahiya A, Sebastian A, Thomas A, George R, Thomas V, Peedicayil A. Endometriosis and malignancy: The intriguing relationship. International Journal of Gynecology & Obstetrics. 2021;**00**:1-7

[11] Nezhat F, Datta MS, Hanson V, Pejovic T, Nezhat C, Nezhat C. The relationship of endometriosis and ovarian malignancy: A review. Fertility and Sterility. 2008;**90**(5):1559-1570

[12] Grandi G, Toss A, Cortesi L, Botticelli L, Volpe A, Cagnacci A. The association between endometriomas and ovarian cancer: Preventive effect of inhibiting ovulation and menstruation during reproductive life. BioMed Research International. 2015;**2015**: 751571

[13] Kuo H-H, Huang C-Y, Ueng S-H, Huang K-G, Lee C-L, Yen C-F. Unexpected epithelial ovarian cancers arising from presumed endometrioma: A 10-year retrospective analysis. Taiwanese Journal of Obstetrics & Gynecology. 2017;**56**:55-61

[14] Kurman RJ, Carcangiu ML, Herrington CS, Young RH. WHO Classification of Tumours of Female Reproductive Organs. Fourth Edition. World Health Organization. Lyon, France: IARC; 2014

[15] Scarfone G, Bergamini A, Noli S, Villa A, Cipriani S, Taccagni G, et al. Characteristics of clear cell ovarian cancer arising from endometriosis: A two center cohort study. Gynecologic Oncology. 2014;**133**(3):480-484

[16] Vercellini P, Viganò P, Buggio L, Makieva S, Scarfone G, Cribiù FM, et al. Perimenopausal management of ovarian endometriosis and associated cancer risk: When is medical or surgical treatment indicated? Best Practice & Research: Clinical Obstetrics & Gynaecology. 2018;**51**:151-168

[17] Moro F, Magoga G, Pasciuto T, Mascilini F, et al. Imaging in gynecological disease (13): Clinical and ultrasound characteristics of endometrioid ovarian cancer. Ultrasound in Obstetrics & Gynecology. 2018;**52**:535-543

[18] Takeuchi M, Matsuzaki K, Uehara H, Nishitani H. Malignant transformation of pelvic endometriosis: MR imaging findings and pathologic correlation. RadioGraphics. 2006;**26**: 407-417

[19] Kim HS, Kim TH, Chung HH, et al. Risk and prognosis of ovarian cancer in women with endometriosis: A meta-analysis. British Journal of Cancer. 2014;**110**:1878-1890

[20] Kvaskoff M, Horne AW, Missmer SA. Informing women with endometriosis about ovarian cancer risk. The Lancet. 2017;**390**(10111): 2433-2434

[21] Sun Y, Liu G. Endometriosis-associated ovarian clear cell carcinoma: A special entity? Journal of Cancer. 2021;**12**(22):6773-6786

[22] Davis M, Rauh-Hain JA, Andrade C, et al. Comparison of clinical outcomes of patients with clear cell and endometrioid ovarian cancer associated with endometriosis to papillary serous carcinoma of the ovary. Gynecologic Oncology. 2014;**132**:760-766

[23] Saavalainen L, Lassus H, But A, Tiitinen A, Härkki P, Gissler M, et al. Risk of gynecologic cancer according to the type of endometriosis. Obstetrics and Gynecology. 2018;**131**(6):1095-1102

[24] Offin M, Chabon JJ, Razavi P, et al. Capturing genomic evolution of lung cancers through liquid biopsy for circulating tumor DNA. Journal of Oncology. 2017;**2017**:4517834. DOI: 10.1155/2017/4517834

[25] Beral V, Doll R, et al. Collaborative group on epidemiological studies of ovarian cancer and oral contraceptives: Collaborative reanalysis of data from 45 epidemiological studies including 23,257 women with ovarian cancer and 87,303 controls. Lancet. 2008;**371**(9609): 303-314

[26] Gaitskell K, Green J, Pirie K, et al. Tubal ligation and ovarian cancer risk in a large cohort: Substantial variation by histological type. International Journal of Cancer. 2016;**138**(5):1076-1084

[27] Melin AS, Lundholm C, Malki N, et al. Hormonal and surgical treatments for endometriosis and risk of epithelial ovarian cancer. Acta Obstetricia et Gynecologica Scandinavica. 2013;**92**: 546-554

[28] Wang KC, Chang WH, Lee WL, et al. An increased risk of epithelial ovarian cancer in Taiwanese women with a new surgico-pathological diagnosis of endometriosis. BMC Cancer. 2014;**14**:831

[29] Pavone ME, Lyttle BM. Endometriosis and ovarian cancer: Links, risks, and challenges faced. International Journal of Women's Health. 2015;**7**:663-667

[30] Stern RC, Dash R, Bentley RC, et al. Malignancy in endometriosis: Frequency and comparison of ovarian and extraovarian types. International Journal of Gynecological Pathology. 2001;**20**:133-139

[31] Rowlands IJ, Nagle CM, Spurdle AB, Webb PM. Gynecological conditions and the risk of endometrial cancer. Gynecologic Oncology. 2011;**123**:537-541

[32] Yu HC, Lin CY, Chang WC, Shen BJ, Chang WP, Chuang CM. Increased association between endometriosis and endometrial cancer. International Journal of Gynecological Cancer. 2015;**25**(3):447-452

[33] Hermens M, van Altena AM, Velthuis I, van de Laar DCM, Bulten J,

van Vliet HAAM, et al. Endometrial cancer incidence in endometriosis and adenomyosis. Cancers. 2021;**13**:4592

[34] Pontikaki A, Sifakis S, Spandidos AD. Endometriosis and breast cancer: A survey of the epidemiological studies. Oncology Letters. 2016;**11**:23-30

[35] Farland LV, Tamimi RM, Eliassen AH, Spiegelman D, Hankinson SE, Chen WY, et al. Laparoscopically confirmed endometriosis and breast cancer in the nurses' health study II. Obstetrics and Gynecology. 2016;**128**(5):1025-1031

[36] Kok Victor C, Tsai H-J, Su C-F, Lee C-K. The risks for ovarian, endometrial, breast, colorectal, and other cancers in women with newly diagnosed endometriosis or adenomyosis. International Journal of Gynecological Cancer. 2015;**25**(6):968-976

[37] Olson JE, Cerhan JR, Janney CA, Anderson KE, Vachon CM, Sellers TA. Postmenopausal cancer risk after self-reported endometriosis diagnosis in the Iowa women's health study. Cancer. 2002;**94**(5):1612-1618

[38] Melin A, Sparén P, Persson I, Bergqvist A. Endometriosis and the risk of cancer with special emphasis on ovarian cancer. Human Reproduction. 2006;**21**(5):1237-1242

[39] Saavalainen L, Lassus H, But A, Tiitinen A, Härkki P, Gissler M, et al. A nationwide cohort study on the risk of non-gynecological cancers in women with surgically verified endometriosis. International Journal of Cancer. 2018;**143**(11):2725-2731

[40] Zahid M, Goldner W, Beseler CL, Rogan EG, Cavalieri EL. Unbalanced estrogen metabolism in thyroid cancer. International Journal of Cancer. 2013;**133**(11):2642-2649

[41] Melin A, Sparén P, Bergqvist A. The risk of cancer and the role of the parity among women with endometriosis. Human Reproduction. 2007;**22**(11): 3021-3026

[42] Claus EB, Calvocoressi L, Bondy ML, Schildkraut JM, Wiemels JL, Wrensch M. Family and personal medical history and risk of meningioma. Journal of Neurosurgery. 2011;**115**(6):1072-1077

[43] Farland LV, Lorrain S, Missmer SA, Dartois L, Cervenka I, Savoye I, et al. Endometriosis and the risk of skin cancer: A prospective cohort study. Cancer Causes & Control. 2017;**28**(10): 1011-1019

[44] Kvaskoff M, Mesrine S, Fournier A, Boutron-Ruault MC, Clavel-Chapelon F. Personal history of endometriosis and risk of cutaneous melanoma in a large prospective cohort of French women. Archives of Internal Medicine. 2007; **167**(19):2061-2065

Chapter 3

Quantitative Imaging Parameters in the Diagnosis of Endometriomas

Paul-Andrei Ștefan, Roxana-Adelina Lupean and Dietmar Tamandl

Abstract

The classic imaging diagnosis of endometriomas encounters multiple limitations, including the subjective evaluation of medical examinations and a similar imaging appearance with other adnexal lesions, especially the functional hemorrhagic cysts. For this reason, a definite diagnosis of endometriomas can be made only by pathological analysis, which reveals particular features in terms of cellularity and biochemical components of their fluid content. It is theorized that these histopathological features can also be reflected in medical images, altering the pixel intensity and distribution, but these changes are too subtle to be assessed by the naked eye. New quantitative imaging evaluations and emerging computer-aided diagnosis techniques can provide a detailed description of image contents that can be furtherly processed by algorithms, aiming to provide a more accurate and non-invasive diagnosis for this disease.

Keywords: computer-aided diagnosis, endometrioma, endometriosis, MRI, texture analysis

1. Introduction

Laparoscopic biopsy of suspicious-looking lesions, followed by histologic confirmation, is the gold standard for diagnosing pelvic endometriosis [1]. The first line imaging of ovarian endometriotic lesions (endometriomas) remains transvaginal ultrasonography (TVUS) which is able, in most situations, to offer sufficient information for adequate preoperative planning [2]. Other diagnostic procedures, such as magnetic resonance imaging (MRI), are used in certain circumstances based on the results of the TVUS and the severity of the symptoms. The pelvic MRI scan provides for full lesion mapping, with a high detection rate for both anterior and, particularly, posterior lesions, whereas TVUS shows lower sensitivity rates [3]. MRI shows higher accuracy for the detection and characterization of endometriotic lesions than other imaging modalities, therefore it is often used to evaluate adnexal masses and monitor treatment response, potentially avoiding the need for a follow-up laparoscopy [4]. Moreover, this method is especially usefull in the detection of deep infiltrating endometriosis, being absolutely required in this subcohort of patients. As with any other imaging modality, the MRI evaluation of endometriosis is limited by the technique itself, but more by the examiner's experience and level of training, since all classic MRI signs of this disease are qualitative and entire subjectively evaluated.

One of the most challenging tasks in the diagnosis of endometriomas is distinguishing these lesions from functional hemorrhagic ovarian cysts (HCs) since they share many both imaging and histological characteristics. To avoid unnecessary surgery, it's critical to correctly distinguish the two lesions [5]. As a result, the difference in imaging between the two entities has a significant impact on the subsequent medical and surgical treatment options [6]. This chapter focuses on the emerging quantitative imaging modalities that can improve the diagnostic and characterization of endometriomas and may aid to distinguish these lesions from HCs.

2. MRI signal intensity measurements

The "T2 shading" sign is currently considered a characteristic MRI finding of endometriomas [7]. This sign refers to a cystic lesion with a high signal on T1-weighted (T1W) sequences and subsequent T2 shortening which results in hypointensity on T2-weighted (T2W) images, as a result of in-lesion hemorrhage and accumulation of blood products and proteins [8, 9].

The "T2 shading" was first described by Togashi and colleagues [10] in 1991, who attributed it high diagnostic value (98% sensitivity and 96% specificity). Following further investigation, more recent studies demonstrated that this sign is not as specific to endometriomas as originally thought, mostly due to the subjective character of the imaging findings [11] and the occurrence of this sign in other ovarian cysts accompanied by bleeding [12–14]. The acknowledgment of these limitations drastically decreased the utility of this sign in further studies (with a sensitivity and specifity as low as 68% and sensitivity and 14.2%, respectively specificity) [11, 12].

It is important to remember that some HCs have a delayed regression and may accumulate blood products, which also leads to a decrease in their intrinsec signal on T2W sequences [14]. However, it is expected that HCs would accumulate f blood products to a lesser degree compared to endometriomas, since they usually regress within a few menstrual cycles and do not exhibit cyclic intra-lesional bleeding. In this regard, Outwater et al. [11] concluded that endometriomas tend to

Author	Year	Sensitivity	Specificity
Dias et al. [15]	2015	73%	93%
Lee et al. [12]	2015	89.8%	14.2%
Outwater et al. [11]	1993	68%	76%
Sugimura et al. [16]	1993	82%	91%
Sugimura et al. [16]	1993	11%	98%
Scout et al. [17]	1994	92%	91%

Table 1.
The diagnostic ability of the "T2 shading" sign for identifying endometriomas.

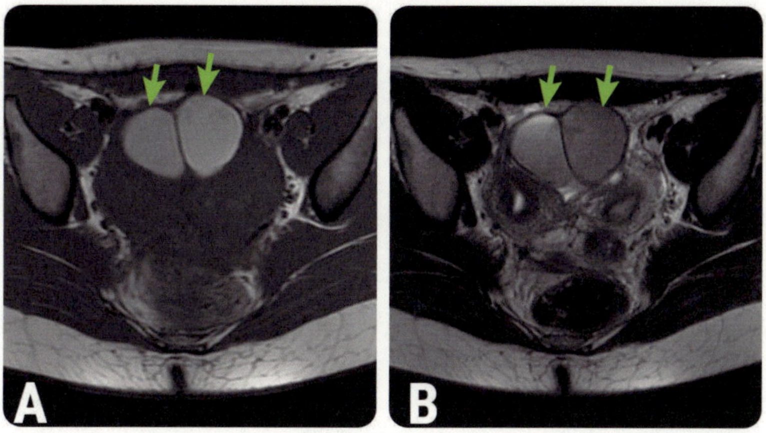

Figure 1.
The magnetic resonance (MRI) representation of the "T2 shading" sign, based on the examination of a patient with two histologically-proven endometriotic lesions. (A) On the axial T1-weighted image, both lesions express similar high-signal intensity (green arrows). (B) On the T2-weighted image, the two lesions express different degrees of signal drop (green arrows).

have higher T1 and lower T2 signal intensities (SI) than HCs, thus creating a more abrupt "shading" phenomenon. However, previous studies did not provide a clear definition of the extent of the signal difference between T1W and T2W sequences, and the degree required for this in order to become a confident diagnostic criterion (**Table 1**). An adequate example of the variation of this signs' appearance is demonstrated in **Figure 1**.

Lately, a small-cohort study [18] aimed to differentiate endometriomas from HCs by quantifying the "T2 shading" sign through signal intensity (SI) measurements made by placing regions of interest (ROIs) within the lesions on T1 and T2 weighted-images (WI). The signal intensity difference was quantified by subtracting SI values between T1 and T2 WI (A = T1 – T2). There were statistically significant differences between the two entities only when comparing T1 SIs ($p = 0.0003$) due to the much higher values obtained by endometriomas, while the T2 SIs were very similar and did not differ significantly ($p = 0.27$). As expected, endometriomas demonstrated a higher loss (median SI loss = 432.95 units) while HCs recorded negative results (median SI loss = −46.8 units). In most cases, the values recorded by HCs on T2 WI were higher than the ones on T1 WI, which could be a consequence of the HCs' blood content being in different stages of degradation and to an overall lesser amount of blood products or protein accumulation (or to a higher percentage of intrinsically present fluid – which is usually not present in endometriomas). These results are in accordance with the early observations of Outwater et al. [11] that were mentioned earlier.

Through the quantitative appreciation of the "shading" sign, using a cut-off for the signal drop of more than 31.3 SI units, endometriomas could be differentiated from HCs with 100% sensitivity and 81.82% specificity. Therefore, this study [18] concluded that the key in identifying endometriomas relies upon a brighter T1 appearance of the lesions, which cannot be always appreciated by the visual evaluation (**Figure 2**). As the proposed measurement technique is rather basic, it could be easily translated into daily clinical practice, possible offering more confidence in the MRI diagnosis of these lesions.

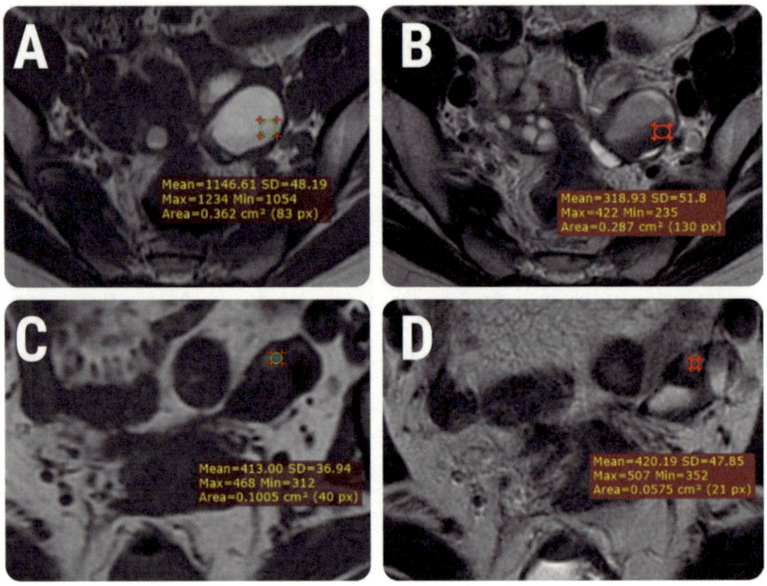

Figure 2.
Quantitative assessment of the "T2 shading" sign in endometriomas and functional hemorrhagic cysts. (A and B) The MRI examination of a 32-year old patient with endometrioma. The difference in signal intensity between (A) T1 (1146.61 units) and (B) T2 (318.93 units) was 827.68 units. (C and D) The MRI examination of a 27-year old patient with an ovarian hemorrhagic cyst. The difference in signal intensity between (C) T1 (413 units) and (D) T2 (420.19 units) was −7.19 units.

3. Diffusion-weighted imaging

MRI incorporates a functional technique known as diffusion-weighted imaging (DWI). DWI sequences provide information about the Brownian motion of water molecules in a tissue [19]. Based on these sequences, apparent diffusion coefficient (ADC) maps can be computed, and together they offer qualitative and quantitative information about tissue density [20]. Tissues that are highly cellular or have cellular swelling show lower water diffusion coefficients which translate to higher SI on DWI sequences and lower values on ADC maps. The ADC value can be quantified as SI values through ROI placement, and can also be used as a marker of cellularity [20]. In recent years, these sequences have evolved as a new tool for the molecular characterization of pathological fluid collections [21]. Technically, the DWI sequences are constructed by acquiring T2-based images at different b-values, through diffusion-sensitizing gradients turned on at various strengths [22]. These b-values reflect the strength and time of the gradients employed to generate such diffusion-weighted images. Subsequently, the diffusion effects are closely linked to the b value [23]. In classic pelvic examinations, ADC maps are automatically generated using all acquired b values. An adequate example is displayed in **Figure 3**. The utility of this technique in differentiating endometriomas from HCs was also investigated in several studies, with contradictory results (**Table 2**).

Overall, the studies conducted by Lee [12] and Balaban [24] showed a statistically significant difference between the ADC values measured in the two groups, while no such difference was observed in a third study conducted by Lupean [18]. Interestingly, in the studies coordinated by Balaban [24] and Lupean [18], the recorded ADC values were higher for HCs than for endometriomas, while Lee [12] obtained opposite results. It is possible that due to the short-living nature of HCs, these lesions do not have the necessary time to build up blood and degradation products, and therefore they produce have a higher motion degree of the water molecules and therefore a lesser decrease of ADC values. However, the differentiation of the two entities based on diffusion

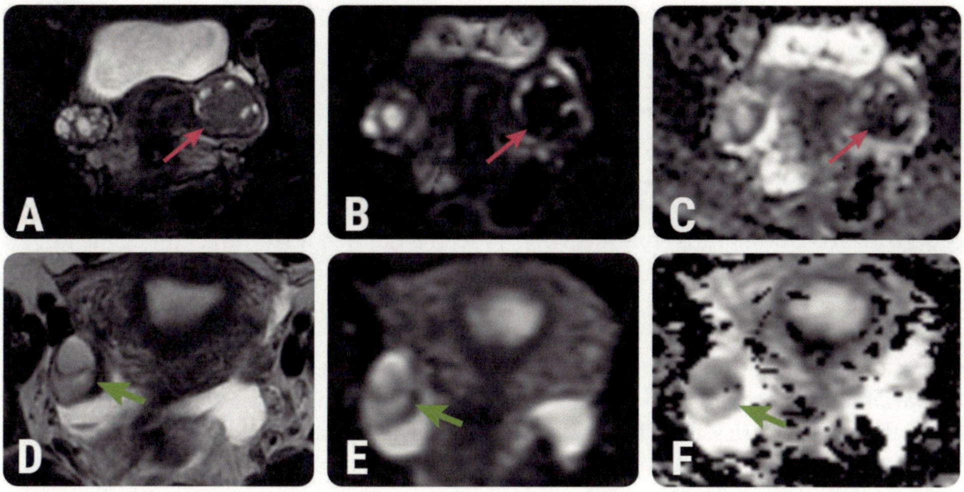

Figure 3.
(A) Axial T2 fat sat, (B) Axial DWI (b = 200), and (C) ADC map of a left-ovarian endometriotic lesion (red arrows). (D) Axial T2, (E) axial DWI, and (F) ADC map of a right-ovarian hemorrhagic cyst (green arrows). There is an obvious lower ADC signal intensity for the endometrioma (red arrow in (C)) than for the hemorrhagic cyst (green arrow in (F)).

Author	Endometriomas		HCs		p-Value	Cut-off	Se	Sp
	n	ADC	n	ADC				
Lee et al. [12]	91	1.06	21	0.73	<0.002	0.849	77.6%	76.2%
Balaban et al. [24]	12	1.84	12	2.70	<0.0001	1.54	100%	92%
Lupean et al. [18]	28	0.964	18	1.001	0.52	—	—	—

n, number of patients; HCs, hemorrhagic cysts; ADC, median ADC values expressed as number × 10^{-3} mm^2/s; cut-off, ADC cut-off value expressed as number × 10^{-3} mm^2/s; p-value, univariate analysis result; Se, sensitivity; Sp, specificity.

Table 2.
The main results that were obtained by studies that focused on the role of differentiating endometriomas from hemorrhagic cysts through apparent diffusion coefficients.

sequences seems unreliable, considering the changing nature of HCs and therefore the variable results obtained in different studies. Therefore, the MRI diffusion techniques may be less suitable for the characterization of ovarian endometriotic lesions.

4. Texture analysis

4.1 Technical considerations

Sometimes the classic imaging features of different types of adnexal lesions may be subtle or overlap, resulting in experts giving the wrong interpretation [25]. For these reasons, in most cases, a definitive diagnosis of an ovarian mass can be made only based on pathological analysis, which raises the patients' risks and healthcare costs.

It is theorized that the several micro and macroscopic histological characteristics of ovarian masses can also be reflected into the background of medical images, but their influence is too subtle to be assessed by the common visual evaluation. Textures represent the intrinsic and intuitive properties of surfaces such as roughness, granulation, and regularity. Texture analysis (TA) is an image processing method based on the extraction and analysis of image-specific parameters that reflect the pixels' distribution patterns and intensity variations [26]. Through these processes, TA provides an objective description of image content by attributing values to several classes of texture parameters. The basic principle of image-based TA is that a pathological process that alters a tissue produces a modified signal, which will, in turn, give textural features different values from those of the normal structure [27].

The standard TA workflow consists of five steps: image segmentation, feature extraction, feature reduction, feature selection, and class prediction. Image segmentation can be performed automatically, semi-automatically, or manually. It consists of incorporating a given structure into a region of interest (ROI). Most often, researchers choose a semi-automatic technique, where a seed is defined near the center of the target lesion and the software automatically delineates the rest of the lesion based on gradient and geometry coordinates. The region or volume of interest could be delineated as a two or three-dimensional structure, the latter being able to provide more information at the cost of higher definition times [19]. However, it was proven that the latter reduces operator variability associated with multislice/volumetric analysis [20]. Therefore, it remains debatable which form will be best suited for clinical implementation. The TA parameters' extraction is performed automatically in almost all available software. The user can, however, adjust several settings regarding the parameters' computation methods (such as the number of bits/pixel and inter-pixel distances). Most software solutions allow the extraction of a large number of texture features (parameters), which can be more difficult to process by researchers that are not familiar with statistical analysis. Therefore, in order to identify the parameters that are most suited to discriminate between groups, several reduction techniques can be available (such as Fisher, Mutual Information, and the probability of classification error and average correlation coefficients) [21]. The number of parameters can be furtherly reduced by univariate analysis (typically the Mann-Whitney U test), or this analysis could be used as the only reduction and selection technique [28]. Class prediction (or the ability of previously-selected texture parameters to distinguish between vectors belonging to different pre-defined groups) can be performed statistically through the receiver operating characteristic analysis or by the use of classifiers (such as k-nearest neighbors algorithm or artificial neural networks) [29]. One of the most often used software for TA-related medical imaging research remains MaZda, which provides build-in functions for feature selection and class prediction [30]. A typical workflow for feature extraction in MaZda is displayed in **Figure 4**.

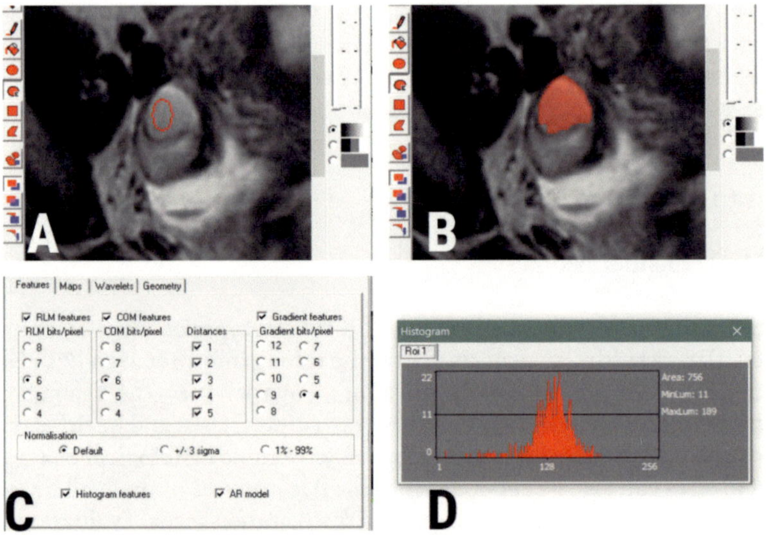

Figure 4.
Workflow within the MaZda software for extracting texture parameters from a T2-weighted MRI image of a patient with an ovarian hemorrhagic cyst. (A) The region of interest (ROI) seed placed by the researcher (red ellipse) and (B) the ROI that was automatically defined by the software. Before feature extraction, parameter settings can be adjusted (C). Histogram representation based on the parameters extracted from the lesion (D).

Texture parameter	Role
Wavelet energy	Measures local variations of pixel intensity [31]
Entropy	Measures the degree of the disorder among pixels within an image; is inversely correlated with uniformity [32]
Sum entropy	Measures the complexity of pixel values distribution [33]
Angular second moment	Directly proportional with the gray level distribution (image uniformity) [34]
Variance	Inversely proportional with image uniformity [35]

Table 3.
A brief description of the MRI-based texture parameters that showed statistically significant results when comparing endometriomas to HCs, based on the study conducted by Lupean et al. [25].

4.2 MRI-based TA for the diagnosis of endometriomas

One study [25] analyzed the texture parameters' ability to distinguish endometriomas from HCs. This study [25] extracted texture features from the internal content of these lesions as seen on T2W. Fourteen parameters showed statistically significant results when comparing the two entities: two variations of the wavelet energy, seven variations of entropy, three of the angular second moment, one of the sum entropy, and the histogram's variance (**Table 3**). Their combined ability was able to differentiate the two entities with a sensitivity of 100% [95% confidence interval (95% CI), 85.8–100%] and a specificity of 100% (95% CI, 71.5–100%).

HCs displayed lower values of wavelet energy, most likely because their content is more homogeneous, resulting in lower signal variation rates [25]. Also, these lesions expressed lower values of the entropy and sum entropy parameters, probably because they do not contain such diverse cell populations and heterogeneous biochemical components compared to endometriomas [36]. Endometriomas on the other hand showed lower values of the angular second moment and higher value of the variance parameter, indicating a lesser uniform content for these lesions (**Figure 5**). These parameters were considered reflections of the heterogeneous content of endometriomas, which otherwise could not be assessed by the usual examinations of the MRI images [25].

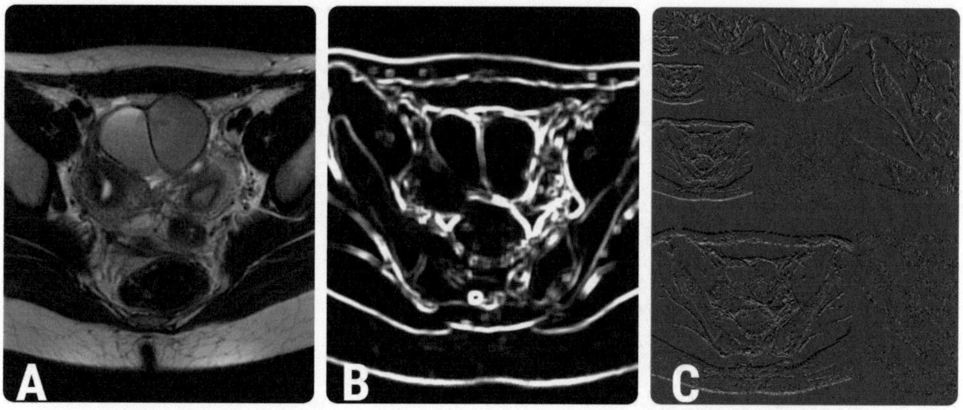

Figure 5.
(A) T2-weighted image of a patient with histologically-proven endometriomas. The texture maps show the distribution of the variance (B) and wavelet energy (C) parameters.

4.3 Ultrasound-based TA for the diagnosis of endometriomas

The ultrasound (US) appearance of endometriomas mainly depends on the time-lapse of blood degradation [37]. Most often, these lesions express a "ground

Author	Year	Se	Sp
Patel et al. [38]	1999	30–95%	49–90%
Mais et al. [39]	1993	84%	90%
Alcázar et al. [40]	1997	88.9%	91%
Van Holsbeke et al. [41]	2010	73%	94%

Table 4.
Studies that evaluated the diagnostic utility of the "ground glass" appearance of endometriomas.

glass" appearance, a feature to which different degrees of accuracy have been attributed over time (**Table 4**).

In practice, the grayscale US of endometriomas and HCs can be very similar, both lesions showing characteristics of different stages of blood degradation, making the distinction difficult [42]. A study [43] showed that 20 texture parameters that were extracted from the US of greyscale images showed statistically significant results when distinguishing endometriomas from HCs. Their combined ability was able to differentiate between the two entities with 100% (95% CI, 88.4–100%) sensitivity and 100% (95% CI, 75.3–100%) [43]. Three parameters were proved to be independent predictors of endometriomas (difference variance, contrast, and the 10th percentile) (**Figure 6**) [43]. The difference of variance parameter measures the variance of the difference of gray level values (reflecting the randomness within an image) [44]. The contrast parameter shows the local variations present in an image, expressing higher values when an image contains a large number of pixels with different gray level values [45]. The study [43] showed that both of these parameters held higher values for HCs than for endometriomas. On the other hand, the 10th percentile showed higher values for endometriomas than for HCs, which signifies that 10% of the pixels within images were distributed under higher values for endometriomas than for HOCs [43]. Even though endometriomas were expected to have a higher degree of echogenic randomness due to a large number of contained elements, HCs displayed higher values for the parameters that mirror these characteristics [43]. This finding is consistent with the literature, which suggests

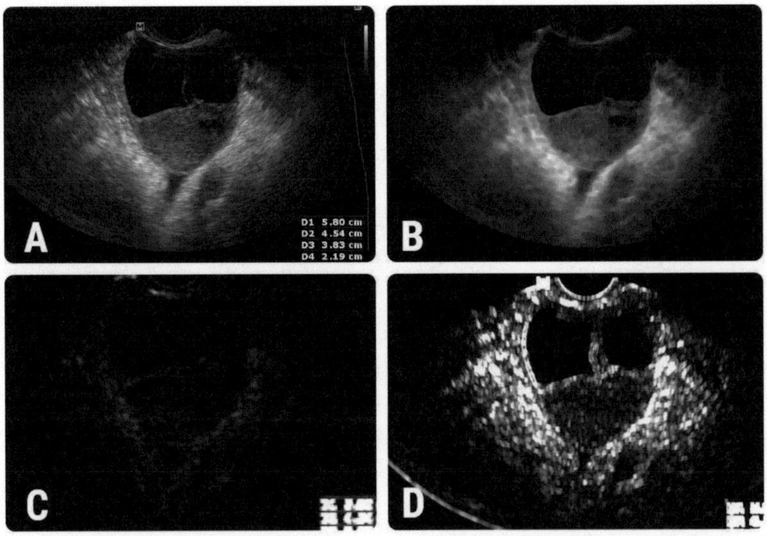

Figure 6.
(A) T2-weighted image of a patient with histologically-proven endometrioma. The texture maps show the distribution of the (B) 10th percentile, (C) contrast, and (D) difference variance parameters.

that HOCs have more complicated and heterogeneous content on TVUS (since they express tiny linear strands and retraction clots more frequently) [46].

5. Conclusion

The current imaging diagnosis of endometriomas encounters several limitations, including a similar appearance to other hemorrhagic adnexal lesions and the subjective nature of the imaging signs considered specific to this disease. Quantitative imaging methods (such as MRI SI measurements and TA) can improve the diagnostic confidence of endometriomas, but the studies validating these methods are certainly required.

Conflict of interest

The authors declare no conflict of interest.

Author details

Paul-Andrei Ştefan[1,2,3], Roxana-Adelina Lupean[1,4]* and Dietmar Tamandl[3]

1 "Iuliu Haţieganu" University of Medicine and Pharmacy, Cluj-Napoca, Romania

2 Radiology and Imaging Department, Cluj County Emergency Clinical Hospital, Cluj-Napoca, Romania

3 Department of Biomedical Imaging and Image-Guided Therapy, Medical University of Vienna, General Hospital of Vienna (AKH), Wien, Österreich

4 Obstetrics and Gynecology Clinic "Dominic Stanca", Cluj County Emergency Hospital, Cluj-Napoca, Romania

*Address all correspondence to: roxanalupean92@gmail.com

References

[1] Siegelman ES, Oliver ER. MR imaging of endometriosis: Ten imaging pearls. Radiographics. 2012;**32**:1675-1691. DOI: 10.1148/rg.326125518

[2] Van den Bosch T, Van Schoubroeck D. Ultrasound diagnosis of endometriosis and adenomyosis: State of the art. Best Practice & Research. Clinical Obstetrics & Gynaecology. 2018;**51**:16-24. DOI: 10.1016/j.bpobgyn.2018.01.013

[3] Kinkel K, Frei KA, Balleyguier C, Chapron C. Diagnosis of endometriosis with imaging: A review. European Radiology. 2006;**16**:285-298. DOI: 10.1007/s00330-005-2882-y

[4] Robinson AJ, Rombauts L, Ades A, Leong K, Paul E, Piessens S. Poor sensitivity of transvaginal ultrasound markers in diagnosis of superficial endometriosis of the uterosacral ligaments. Journal of Endometriosis and Pelvic Pain Disorders. 2018;**10**:10-17. DOI: 10.1177/2284026518767259

[5] Kim H-J, Lee S-Y, Shin YR, Park CS, Kim K. The value of diffusion-weighted imaging in the differential diagnosis of ovarian lesions: A meta-analysis. PLoS One. 2016;**11**:e0149465. DOI: 10.1371/journal.pone.0149465

[6] Tanase Y, Kawaguchi R, Takahama J, Kobayashi H. Factors that differentiate between endometriosis-associated ovarian cancer and benign ovarian endometriosis with mural nodules. Magnetic Resonance in Medical Sciences. 2018;**17**:231-237. DOI: 10.2463/mrms.mp.2016-0149

[7] Foti PV, Attinà G, Spadola S, Caltabiano R, Farina R, Palmucci S, et al. MR imaging of ovarian masses: Classification and differential diagnosis. Insights Into Imaging. 2016;7:21-41. DOI: 10.1007/s13244-015-0455-4

[8] Glastonbury CM. The Shading Sign. Radiology. 2002;**224**:199-201. DOI: 10.1148/radiol.2241010361

[9] Siegelman ES, Outwater EK. Tissue characterization in the female pelvis by means of MR imaging. Radiology. 1999;**212**:5-18. DOI: 10.1148/radiology.212.1.r99jl455

[10] Togashi K, Nishimura K, Kimura I, Tsuda Y, Yamashita K, Shibata T, et al. Endometrial cysts: Diagnosis with MR imaging. Radiology. 1991;**180**:73-78. DOI: 10.1148/radiology.180.1.2052726

[11] Outwater E, Schiebler ML, Owen RS, Schnall MD. Characterization of hemorrhagic adnexal lesions with MR imaging: Blinded reader study. Radiology. 1993;**186**:489-494. DOI: 10.1148/radiology.186.2.8421756

[12] Lee NK, Kim S, Kim KH, Suh DS, Kim TU, Han GJ, et al. Diffusion-weighted magnetic resonance imaging in the differentiation of endometriomas from hemorrhagic cysts in the ovary. Acta Radiologica. 2016;**57**:998-1005. DOI: 10.1177/0284185115609805

[13] Corwin MT, Gerscovich EO, Lamba R, Wilson M, McGahan JP. Differentiation of ovarian endometriomas from hemorrhagic cysts at MR imaging: Utility of the T2 dark spot sign. Radiology. 2014;**271**:126-132. DOI: 10.1148/radiol.13131394

[14] Kanso HN, Hachem K, Aoun NJ, Haddad-Zebouni S, Klein-Tomb L, Atallah D, et al. Variable MR findings in ovarian functional hemorrhagic cysts. Journal of Magnetic Resonance Imaging. 2006;**24**:356-361. DOI: 10.1002/jmri.20640

[15] Dias JL, Veloso Gomes F, Lucas R, Cunha TM. The shading sign: Is it exclusive of endometriomas? Abdominal Imaging. 2015;**40**:2566-2572. DOI: 10.1007/s00261-015-0465-1

[16] Sugimura K, Okizuka H, Imaoka I, Kaji Y, Takahashi K, Kitao M, et al. Pelvic endometriosis: Detection and diagnosis with chemical shift MR imaging. Radiology. 1993;**188**:435-438. DOI: 10.1148/radiology.188.2.8327693

[17] Scoutt LM, McCarthy SM, Lange R, Bourque A, Schwartz PE. MR evaluation of clinically suspected adnexal masses. Journal of Computer Assisted Tomography. 1994;**18**:609-618. DOI: 10.1097/00004728-199407000-00019

[18] Lupean R-A, Ștefan P-A, Lebovici A, Csutak C, Rusu GM, Mihu CM. Differentiation of endometriomas from hemorrhagic cysts at magnetic resonance: The role of quantitative signal intensity measurements. Current Medical Imaging. 2021;**17**:524-531. DOI: 10.2174/1573405616999201027211132

[19] Agostinho L, Horta M, Salvador JC, Cunha TM. Benign ovarian lesions with restricted diffusion. Radiologia Brasileira. 2019;**52**:106-111. DOI: 10.1590/0100-3984.2018.0078

[20] Lupean R-A, Ștefan P-A, Feier DS, Csutak C, Ganeshan B, Lebovici A, et al. Radiomic analysis of MRI images is instrumental to the stratification of ovarian cysts. Journal of Personalized Medicine. 2020;**10**:E127. DOI: 10.3390/jpm10030127

[21] Mayerhoefer ME, Breitenseher M, Amann G, Dominkus M. Are signal intensity and homogeneity useful parameters for distinguishing between benign and malignant soft tissue masses on MR images? Objective evaluation by means of texture analysis. Magnetic Resonance Imaging. 2008;**26**:1316-1322. DOI: 10.1016/j.mri.2008.02.013

[22] DWI. Questions and Answers in MRI. Availble from: http://mriquestions.com/making-a-dw-image.html [Accessed: November 3, 2021]

[23] b-value diffusion. Questions and Answers in MRI. Available from: http://mriquestions.com/what-is-the-b-value.html [Accessed: November 3, 2021]

[24] Balaban M, Idilman IS, Toprak H, Unal O, Ipek A, Kocakoc E. The utility of diffusion-weighted magnetic resonance imaging in differentiation of endometriomas from hemorrhagic ovarian cysts. Clinical Imaging. 2015;**39**:830-833. DOI: 10.1016/j.clinimag.2015.05.003

[25] Lupean R-A, Ștefan P-A, Csutak C, Lebovici A, Măluțan AM, Buiga R, et al. Differentiation of endometriomas from ovarian hemorrhagic cysts at magnetic resonance: The role of texture analysis. Medicina (Kaunas, Lithuania). 2020;**56**:E487. DOI: 10.3390/medicina56100487

[26] Larroza A, Bodí V, Moratal D. Texture analysis in magnetic resonance imaging: Review and considerations for future applications. In: Assessment of Cellular and Organ Function and Dysfunction Using Direct and Derived MRI Methodologies. London, UK: InTechOpen; 2016

[27] Morris DT. An evaluation of the use of texture measurements for the tissue characterisation of ultrasonic images of in vivo human placentae. Ultrasound in Medicine & Biology. 1988;**14**:387-395. DOI: 10.1016/0301-5629(88)90074-9

[28] Csutak C, Ștefan P-A, Lenghel LM, Moroșanu CO, Lupean R-A, Șimonca L, et al. Differentiating high-grade gliomas from brain metastases at magnetic resonance: The role of texture analysis of the peritumoral zone. Brain Sciences. 2020;**10**:E638. DOI: 10.3390/brainsci10090638

[29] Stefan P-A, Puscas ME, Csuak C, Lebovici A, Petresc B, Lupean R, et al. The utility of texture-based classification of different types of ascites on magnetic resonance. Journal of BUON. 2020;**25**:1237-1244

[30] Strzelecki M, Szczypinski P, Materka A, Klepaczko A. A software tool for automatic classification and segmentation of 2D/3D medical images. Nuclear Instruments and Methods in Physics Research A. 2013;**702**:137-140

[31] Livens S. Wavelets for texture analysis, an overview. In: Proceedings of the 6th International Conference on Image Processing and its Applications. Dublin, Ireland: IET - Institution of Engineering and Technology; 14-17 July 1997. pp. 581-585

[32] Zhao H, Feng X, Chen Y, Zhao S, Xiao P. Entropy-based texture analysis and feature extraction of urban street trees in the spatial frequency domain. In: Proceedings of the Sixth International Symposium on Multispectral Image Processing and Pattern Recognition. Yichang, China: Society of Photo-Optical Instrumentation Engineers (SPIE); 30 October–1 November 2009. Vol. 7495. p. 749513

[33] Jernigan ME, D'Astous F. Entropy-based texture analysis in the spatial frequency domain. IEEE Transactions on Pattern Analysis and Machine Intelligence. 1984;**6**:237-243

[34] Texture Analysis Using Co-Occurrence Matrix. Available from: https://www.massey.ac.nz/~{}mjjohnso/notes/59731/presentations/texture.pdf [Accessed: August 12, 2021]

[35] Writh A. Texture Analysis. Available from: http://www.cyto.purdue.edu/cdroms/micro2/content/education/wirth06.pdf [Accessed: August 13, 2021]

[36] Bibbo M, Wood MD, Fitzpatrick BT. Peritoneal washings and ovary. In: Wilbur D, editor. Comprehensive Cyto-Pathology E-Book. Amsterdam, The Netherlands: Elsevier Health Sciences; 2014. pp. 291-301

[37] Collins BG, Ankola A, Gola S, McGillen KL. Transvaginal US of endometriosis: Looking beyond the endometrioma with a dedicated protocol. Radiographics. 2019;**39**:1549-1568. DOI: 10.1148/rg.2019190045

[38] Patel MD, Feldstein VA, Chen DC, Lipson SD, Filly RA. Endometriomas: Diagnostic performance of US. Radiology. 1999;**210**:739-745. DOI: 10.1148/radiology.210.3.r99fe61739

[39] Mais V, Guerriero S, Ajossa S, Angiolucci M, Paoletti AM, Melis GB. The efficiency of transvaginal ultrasonography in the diagnosis of endometrioma. Fertility and Sterility. 1993;**60**:776-780. DOI: 10.1016/S0015-0282(16)56275-X

[40] Alcázar JL, Laparte C, Jurado M, Lopez-Garcia G. The role of transvaginal ultrasonography combined with color velocity imaging and pulsed Doppler in the diagnosis of endometrioma. Fertility and Sterility. 1997;**67**:487-491. DOI: 10.1016/S0015-0282(97)80074-X

[41] Van Holsbeke C, Van Calster B, Guerriero S, Savelli L, Paladini D, Lissoni AA, et al. Endometriomas: Their ultrasound characteristics. Ultrasound in Obstetrics & Gynecology. 2010;**35**:730-740. DOI: 10.1002/uog.7668

[42] Batur A, Yavuz A, Ozgokce M, Bora A, Bulut MD, Arslan H, et al. The utility of ultrasound elastography in differentiation of endometriomas and hemorrhagic ovarian cysts. Journal of Medical Ultrasonics. 2016;**43**:395-400. DOI: 10.1007/s10396-016-0701-5

[43] Ştefan R-A, Ştefan P-A, Mihu CM, Csutak C, Melincovici CS, Crivii CB, et al. Ultrasonography in the differentiation of endometriomas from hemorrhagic ovarian cysts: The role of texture analysis. Journal of Personalized Medicine. 2021;**11**:611. DOI: 10.3390/jpm11070611

[44] Durgamahanthi V, Christaline JA, Edward AS. GLCM and GLRLM based texture analysis: Application to brain cancer diagnosis using histopathology images. In: ; Dash SS, Das S, Panigrahi BK. Intelligent Computing and Applications. Singapore: Springer; 2020; pp. 691-706

[45] Biomedical Informatics 260. Computational Feature Extraction: Texture Features Lecture 6 David Paik. Available from: https://docplayer.net/188454072-Biomedical-informatics-260-computational-feature-extraction-texture-features-lecture-6-david-paik-phd-spring-2019.html [Accessed: May 26, 2021]

[46] Rezvani M. Nonneoplastic ovarian lesions: Endometrioma. In: Shaaban AM, Menias CO, Tubay MS, editors. Diagnostic Imaging: Gynecology. 2nd ed. Amsterdam, The Netherlands: Elsevier; 2015. p. 190

Chapter 4

Potential Therapeutic Options and Perspectives for Alleviation of Endometrial Estrogen Dominance and Progesterone Resistance in Endometriosis

Manuela Cristina Russu

Abstract

Endometriosis is a chronic disease, influenced by internal and external environment, with long duration from intrauterine life with acme during childbearing, when it is associated to chronic pelvic pains, and infertility/subfertility. DNA hypermethylation of endometrial promoter PRs *Hox genes* and DNA hypomethylation of promoter ERβ *gene* is a possible explanation of estrogen dominance, progressive loss of progesterone signaling, followed by progesterone resistance in ectopic, and progesterone attenuance in eutopic endometrium, for failure of hormone therapy (HT), repeated recurrences after surgery, cancers after long time evolution. Animal models, human trials demonstrated progesterone (P4) and progestins influences over progression of disease pathological characteristics, associated to endometrial ER, PR aberrant expressions: ERα loss, and abnormal PRB/PRA *ratio*. P4 supplementation before mice induced-endometriosis protected from PRs depletion, action that can be translated in women according to the difference of 7 to 12 years between histologic onset and clinical symptoms/signs, parallel to progressive loss of PRs and PR-mediated signaling in ectopic and eutopic endometria. The animal studies have shown that a DNA methylation inhibitor alleviates lesion growth, and induces PRs target gene expression restoration. Continuous/extended contraceptives, dienogest-a new progestin, GnRH agonists/antagonists, aromatase inhibitors, SERM, SPRM, combinated molecules are therapeutic options/perspectives aiming restoration endometrial estrogen-progesterone balance, without disease's cure. HT may be active alone, or surgery associated.

Keywords: endometriosis, estrogen dominance, progesterone resistance/attenuance, timing, progesterone/progestins, DNA methylation inhibition

1. Introduction

Urgent innovations are demanded in endometriosis management, which should start by deeper undestanding of disease core features, with disease different phenotypes and idiosyncrasies. Endometriosis, a chronic inflammatory and immune disease, dependent on environement factors, genes- *Hox* genes code (HOXA10/HOXA11), epigenetics, and ovarian steroid hormones, with their receptors and coregulators in the eutopic endometrium and ectopic sites, was demonstrated to have a long duration of progress from intrauterine life, latency in childhood, and acme during reproductive years [1–3] with reappearance in postmenopause when hormone replacement therapy, or even without [4]. This fact permits therapeutic intervention to correct endometrial abnormal functions during menstrual cycle, to prepare decidua receptivity for successful egg implantation in women with minimal or mild to moderate endometriosis, in order to avoid the severe stages, and lack of response to therapy, considering that progesterone resistance is an acquired property of eutopic endometrium [5]. The therapeutic aims are to prevent, or at least to stop the progressive damages induced by ectopic endometriotic lesions in the uterus, entire genital tract, and in extra-uterine sites by the endometrial mezenchymal stromal/stem/progenitor cells with their specific migratory, adhesive, and invasive properties, with their genome changes when are outside the uterus, to influence the self- protected endometriotic lesions [6] and to ensure a normal eutopic endometrial cycle functioning, with normal ovarian steroid hormones receptors distribution during menstrual cycle. The aims can be individually accomplished if therapy is started from early stages of illness, by moving from pure hormonal therapy to drug combination, or novel molecules- SERMs, SPRMs which can escape the disrupted homeostatic mechanisms characteristic for endometriosis [7].

One may propose and discuss a perspective "timing" of endometriosis treatment, to maintain or for an early restoration of endometrial estrogen- progesterone receptors natural balance [8] being recognized a still delay in diagnosis, and treatment [9] delay that permits the evolution of genital damages by progressing endometriosis, and in time the risk of atypical endometriosis, and cancers which is very difficult to be assessed clinically, without specific biochemical markers [10].

The incidence of endometriosis of one case in 10 women of reproductive age [11, 12] or around 17% [13] is increasing when one assseses infertility and chronic pelvic pains - up to 50% [14] respectively up to 60% [15] recently being estimated 176 million women worldwide, making endometriosis as common as diabetes mellitus [16].

There are three distinct forms of disease according to ectopic sites of endometrial-like tissue location (peritoneal, ovarian and rectovaginal endometriosis), each of them being associated with specific symptoms, although dysmenorrhea, and chronic non-menstrual pelvic pains, dyschezia, dyspareunia are the most frecquent [17]. The literature makes some differences regarding the score of endometriosis, namely the ENZIAN classification/score describes superficial (less than 1 mm), intermediate (2 to 4 mm), deep (greater than or equal to 5 mm), and very deep implants (greater than 10 mm) [18]. The ENZIAN score was proposed of the revised American Society of Reproductive Medicine score (1996) [19], which was demonstrated to be less adequate to clinics, and the ENZIAN score was recently reviewed by experts in imagistic and surgical diagnosis [20]. So endometriosis has a similarity to oncology with 4 stages of evolution, with the difference of missing nuclear atypia [21] but with possible evolution to malignancy in 1% cases [1, 22] or further it may be associated to hematopoietic and breast cancer (HR of 1,3–95% CI 1.1–1.4, in Swidish women) [23] and ovarian cancer, – OR of 1.73, (95% CI: 1.10-2.71) on a pool of women from different continents- Australia, Canada, Denmark, USA, during 10 years (1989–1999) with previous endometriosis [24]. The natural history of endometriosis is uncertain, e.g. it is not known whether superficial peritoneal endometriosis (SPE) can progress to become another subtype, regress spontaneously, or whether disease progression (or lack of treatment) can lead to problems with infertility, and there is poor correlation between pain severity and the amount, location, and subtype of the ectopic lesions [16].

The literature does not mention a conclusive noninvasive diagnostic available tool to allow early detection of endometriosis, the delay in detection being of 7–12 years of latency from symptoms onset to the definitive diagnosis, and even in the best medical centres the full extent of the disease may be unknown [25] and up to 2017 it was not identified any fully validated, symptom-based, patient- reported questionnaire for endometriosis screening in adult women with potential endometriosis [26]. One must think to endometriosis in adolescent girls with family history, abnormal characteristics of menstrual cycles with the aim to avoid the structural and functional abnormalities progression induced in women's endometrial genes - mainly *Hox* codes for steroid hormones receptors, ligands, and co-regulators.

The next pages will discuss concepts, theories or hypothesis of potential therapeutic options and perspectives for prevention, normalization or restoration the endometrial estrogen- progesterone balance, and their receptors in the epithelium and stroma, because many years there were recommended ovarian supressing drugs, and surgery.

2. Endometrial phenotypes in endometriosis

The interest for diagnosis and therapeutic success connected to side effects, limitations and failure rate of different classes of medication, and high risks of recurrence after surgery or medication discontinuation imposed the analysis of endometrium phenotypes, proliferative and differention *in vitro* capacities of stromal cells from ectopic lesions of peritoneum, ovaries, and deeply infiltrating endometriosis in comparison to the same structures of normal women, using the new techniques as contrast microscopy, immunocytochemistry, functional bioassays [27] and RT- qPCR of endometrial genes.

The study of Burney et al. [28] analyzed eutopic and ectopic endometria comparative to non ill women, and it was demonstrated a molecular phenotype of attenuated progesterone response within eutopic endometrium, from the dysregulation of numerous genes which are progesterone regulated, and the progesterone resistant phenotype is more frecquent in ectopic endometrium comparative to non-ill cases. This condition is associated to a pro-inflammatory phenotype [29, 30] which increases both estrogen dominance, and progesterone resistance. The eutopic endometrium of ill women has an attenuate response to P4 because estrogen-responsive genes are not suppressed in their stromal cells in early secretory phase of menstrual cycle comparative to normal [28, 31, 32]. The British and Italian doctors' conclusion [29] was that endometriotic cell lines, and stromal eutopic endometrial cells in ill-women are lossing the capacities of differentiation, and respectively of deciadualisation, aspects that explain cells capacities for proliferation and survival in the ectopic environment, and high infertility/subfertility rates. Deep endometriosis appears to be a special type, because predominance of PR less active isoform (PR-A) over the full length, due to epigenetic abnormalities affecting PR gene transcription, associated to oxidative stress, facts that induce a condition of more resistant to size regression upon medical treatments [7].

3. Concepts on endometrial peculiarities, as a steroid hormones target in endometriosis. Estrogen dominance. Progesterone resistance. Progesterone attenuance

The efficacy of endometriosis therapies may be improved by dissecting the unique molecular properties of eutopic and ectopic endometria compared to normal endometrium. At first glance, the terms "estrogen dominance" and "progesterone resistance" appear to describe opposite sides of the same coin [6]. Endometrial Progesterone Resistance is described since many years [33] as there are other hormones resistance, being first named as "Pseudocorpus Luteum Insufficiency" [34] meaning that endometrium is not able to respond to bioavailable P4 plasma levels inbetween normal limits. In non-ill women E2 induces epithelial proliferation to build endometrial thickness during the proliferative phase of the menstrual cycle, then P4 inhibits E2-induced proliferation and allows stromal cells to begin decidualization during the secretory phase [35] in order to prepare the stroma to become receptive to blastocyst invasion during "window of receptivity/implantation" in normal, fertile women [36].

3.1 Dysregulation of endometrial steroid hormones receptors in endometriosis

The molecular mechanism triggered by ovarian steroid hormones in endometrium is well known: steroid hormones link to specific nuclear (ERα, ERβ; PRA, PR-B, with specific ratios between them), cytoplasmic (ERβ), and membrane receptors (non- canonical G protein-coupled estrogen receptor (GPER) [37] and PGRMC-1 and PGRMC-2), which are able to bind to the promoter of the target genes, being up- or down- regulated by their co-activators (SRC-1, SRC-2, SRC-3 for estrogen receptors- ER) or downstream effectors (TGFβ, Dickkopf-1, retinoic acid, c-*myc*, *etc.* for progesterone receptors- PRs) [28] and influence endometrial cells proliferation and differentiation [38]. Endometrial repair after menstruation, proliferation and/or differentiation processes are dysregulated in endometriosis when menstrual reflux with endometrial stromal and epithelial glands cells with their exosomes migrate, adhere and invade peritoneal surface and/or other ectopic sites, associated to waves of inflammation (by systemic and local reactive responses to the presence of endometrial debris), neuro- angiogenesis and neuroinflammation, and aberrant scar formation through fibrosis and adherences (possible a self-protection mechanism for ectopic lesion, as in chronic infections) at every ovarian cycle (different from normal endometrium restoration after each menstrual cycle). All these events are genetic controlled, epigenetic changed by hyper (for PR promoter) or hypomethylation (for ERβ) of DNA steroid hormones receptors promoters [39–41]. When the tightly regulated balance of epithelial- stromal P4 and E2 signaling is lost, P4 resistance and E2 dominance are prone to ensue, as in endometriosis [6]. P4 resistance may lead to both increased lesion growth and a non-receptive endometrium, and actually one speaks also about progesterone attenuated response in eutopic endometrium, which is associated to infertilty/subfertility. Estrogen dominance, progesterone resistance and progesterone attenuance in the ectopic and eutopic endometrium are explained by the dysregulation of estrogen and progesterone receptors their genes (*ESR1* and *ESR2*) [32]; a single gene- *PRG* for PRs) [42] with their micro-RNA (miRNA) –the cells' critical regulators for development, and physiology, their mis-expression being associated to pathology [43].

When dysregulation condition persists it leads to both increased lesion growth and progression to a superior stage, and a non-receptive endometrium. P4 acts on stromal cells of the normal endometrium, inducing paracrine factor(s), and they induce the expression of the enzyme 17β-hydroxysteriod dehydrogenase type 2 (17β-HSD-2) for metabolization of E_2 to estrone (E_1), in the epithelial cells, and cell proliferation arrest. Excess E2 with Estrogen Dominance, and Progesterone Resistance are well documented in ectopic endometrium with aberrant levels of ERs and changed ER-α/ ER β *ratio*, where the genes analyses have proved to become an acquired property, through their migration and exposure process to peritoneal environement [5]. ER-α and ER- β have essential roles in establishment and progression of ectopic lesions [32]. ERβ is excessively expressed in stromal cells of the ectopic lesions, versus non-ill women, fact due to hypomethylation of ERβ promoter, which contributes to low ER-α expression in ectopic endometrium [41, 44]. ERβ protein net -work together with SRC-1 coactivator isoform with which it cooperates, may have a cytoplasmic, non-genomic action in endometriosis as Han SJ, Jung SY, Wu SP, et al. discovered [44] (**Figure 1**).

Eutopic endometrium may prove the same endometrial dominance and progesterone resistance, but after some years of disesease evolution, being described cases with initial progesterone attenuance in eutopic endometrium and progesterone resistance in the ectopic sites, usually in deep endometriosis [28]. It is documented a local increased synthesis of estrogen [45, 46] not a systemic high level [47] through the presence of the enzymens (aromatase, and 17β-hydroxysteroid dehydrogenase-1, 17β-HSD-1) [48, 49] and a blunted response to progesterone in eutopic and ectopic endometrium, P4 serum levels being similar to non- ill women [45]. In human and experimental mice the ER-α content may be normal in eutopic endometrium, as in non ill women, but ER β are increased in both epithelial and stromal endometrial cells of eutopic and ectopic sites, as PRs levels are reduced in eutopic endometrium and PRs are lost in ectopic sites [44]. A recent analyses of ERs in deep endometriosis revealed that ER-α is a subtype for this condition [50] ER-α levels being predictive for symptoms severity, and for responses to treatment [51]. Progesterone attenuance of eutopic endometrium is connected to altered endometrial receptivity in the "window of receptivity/implantation" and to a significant reduction of implantation rate in ill-patients trying *in vitro* fertilization, due to stromal cells impair decidualization proved by a reduction of nearly 2-fold in IGFBP-1, and of leukemia inhibitory factor (LIF) [52] and to reduction/dysregulation of P4 target genes during the "window of receptivity/implantation", time when normally, the endometrium is exposed to the highest levels of P4 [53] as it is strikingly down-regulated *glycodelin*- the prototype progesterone-responsive gene, in eutopic endometrium of ill-women compared to non-ill [53, 54]. LIF low levels are an intrisic glandular dysfunction, induced by the gland-specific transcription factor Forkhead box A2 (FOXA2) low level [55, 56] also a P4 gene target. There are contradictions on the status of ERs and PRs in ectopic endometrium – an ERs increased expression, or others show reduced expression of both ERα and ERβ

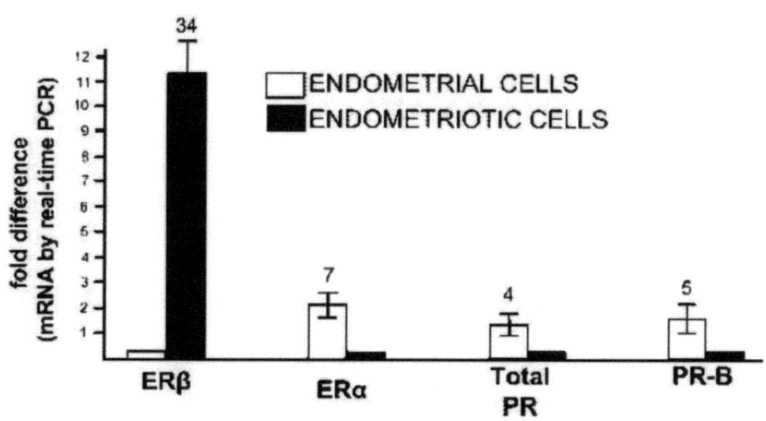

Figure 1.
Role of ER-β in endometriosis. microRNA levels of steroids in primary stromal cells isolated from endometrium and endometriosis (n = 8 patients in each category). Comparable in vivo differences were also observed between whole tissues of endometrium and endometriosis Legend: ER: estrogen receptor; PR: progesterone receptor; real time-PCR: polymerase chain reaction (adapted from Bulun et al. [45]: open acces).

[57–59] and lower levels of PRs [5, 60]. The eutopic endometrium has an attenuate answer to P4, the isoform PR- B is not expressed in patients' endometrium, being only the isoform PR-A, because progesterone-responsive genes are not deleted in eutopic endometrium in comparison to normal women in the early secretory phase of cycle [28–32], a normal PR-A/PR-B *ratio* is very important in endometrial function. One may consider that the relative differences between studies regarding the PR isoforms loss in ectopic and eutopic endometrium may be explained by stage of disease, type of lesion and cells, and method of analysis.

Previous studies [32] demonstrated in experimental mice that high levels of ERα are driving proliferation, adhesion and angiogenesis in ectopic tissue, and also modulate inflammation, and ERβ prevents apoptosis and enhance invasion, proliferation, adhesion, and inflammation to stimulate the growth of ectopic lesion, so both isoforms might sinergistically contribute to regulation of proliferation, adhesion, and inflammation in endometriotic lesion. These discrepant findings are explained by the differences in study design, patient selection criteria, cycle stage, and endometriosis type and stage. Similar to these contradictory results on endometrial steroid hormones receptors is the situation with miRNA indentification by real-time quantitative reverse transcription-polymerase chain reaction (real time qRT-PCR) in normal endometrium, eutopic and ectopic sites, connected to mi-RNA upregulation (over expression) or down regulation (under expression) in eutopic and in different ectopic areas (peritoneal, ovarian), and some are "mis-expressed" endometriosis [61]. There are differences between authors, with conflicting reports on whether or not miRNA expression was influenced by the menstrual cycle phases, endometrial cell type, miRNA type, level in ectopic/eutopic tissue, and stage of disease.

3.2 High micro-heterogeneity of endometrial steroid hormones receptors signaling in endometriosis

Normal endometrium is containing large quantities of distinct stromal cells with abundant estrogen-induced PRs, which influence glandular epithelial cell proliferation and differentiation, and protect against carcinogenic transformation, when PRA/PRB are in a proper *ratio* to ensure normal P4 response. PRA and PRB are members of a superfamily of almost 50 ligand-activated nuclear transcription factors [62]. *In-vitro* studies suggest that the two PR isoforms differ functionally, and that their relative expression in a target cell may determine the nature and magnitude of response to P4. The two isoforms are in comparable levels expressed in proliferative phase, but in the mid- secretory only PR- B is present in the epithelial glands, PR-A is predominantly present in the stroma throughout the cycle. It is a homogeneity in the relative expression in PR-A and PR-B in adjacent cells within the same tissue compartment, and a heterogeneity between glands, observed under some circumstances in the endometrium functionalis, suggesting that PR isoforms down-regulation by P4 is asynchronous, and between the glands of the basalis and functionalis of the endometrium implying region specific responses to hormonal stimuli [63].

A recent European study on deep endometriosis [64] showed a high variability of ERα and PR distribution in the same gland, among distinct glands of the same sample, and among distinct patients receiving the same treatment. Luminal epithelial height variability was primarily due to epithelial cells heterogeneity in a gland, secondarily to the glands randomaly evaluated on the same section, and tertiary to the patient category. The heterogeneity of ERα and PR distribution in the same women could explain why endocrine treatments are unable to cure deep endometrios. The cause of heterogeneity in endometriotic tissues is difficult to be ascertain, one hypothesis being the DNA methylation of the steroid hormones [65] or of their promoters [39, 40] or an abnormal proteolysis of steroid hormones chaperons [66], the co-chaperons are required by PR for signaling uterine cycles and implantation [67].

Mice induced endometriosis demonstrated a high inter-animal variation in the levels of ERs, PRs, in ectopic endometrium vs. controls; with variable levels by almost 100-fold within the same lesion, and with differences between two lesions from the same animal [68] aspect called "micro-heterogeneity". The changes are tissue intrinsic, and some researchers propose that the variable outcomes in hormonal therapy for endometriosis could be possibly due to heterogeneity or polymorphism in the expression of steroid hormone receptors in the ectopic endometrium [68] or in all endometrial locations- eutopic, and ectopic, being known the heterogeneity of PRs in glands, and the homogeneity of PR isoforms in stroma of normal human endometrium [63] making the magnitude in response, the attenuance, and the resistance in response to P4, independently to the serum levels of P4 [69]. This intrinsic biologic alteration of eutopic endometrium explains the missing differences in endometrial thickness, and histology –respectively luteal differentiation, or epithelial integrin expression at the lower mid-luteal serum progesterone level (as 3–4 ng/ml) in programmed cycles of physiological and subphysiological exogenous progesterone replacement in GnRH agonist-suppressed healthy volunteers. One may consider that these results are an answer to the questions whether the abnormalities of eutopic endometrium in early secretory phase suggestive of attenuated progesterone response in the transition from proliferative to secretory phase are due to lower level of circulation or local bioavailable progesterone or to the changes in endometrial transcriptome, with dysregulation of progesterone- regulated genes.

3.3 Nuclear receptor coregulators in the modulation of progesterone and estrogen signaling in endometriosis

Endocrinologic literature presents different series of nuclear receptors coregulators,- proteins that intervene to modify chromatin structure and regulate large-scale gene transcription programs by forming large complexes with the nuclear receptors of the target cells [70]. In the female genital tract the *PRG* and *ESR1* are critically regulated by a family of regulatory proteins named steroid receptor coactivators (SRCs) - SRC-1, SRC-2, and SRC-3, the first nuclear receptors coregulators are involved in the balance between E2 and P4 in human endometrium. SRC-1 down regulates P4 target genes in the epithelium, and up regulates them in the stroma; SRC-2 is necessary for human endometrial stromal cells decidualisation [71] for P4 signaling and for ESR1 signaling; the transcriptomic analysis revealed that 50% of SRC-2-regulated genes are also regulated by P4 [72] and it is critical for murine uterine function; ablation of SRC-2 induces partial loss of decidualisation and infertility, and both SRCs ablation induces complete loss of decidualisation [73, 74].

4. Potential therapeutic options to maintain/restore endometrial normal estrogen-progesterone signaling in endometriosis

Presently pharmacotherapy mainly with hormones (Hormone Therapy- HT) and surgery are two cornerstones in endometriosis management. Surgery with histological confirmation of ectopic endometrial glands and stroma remains the gold standard for diagnosis [75, 76] surgery being generally reserved for patients who fail medical therapy, or who desire pregnancy, being usually performed by laparoscopy [77, 78]. Surgery is able to eliminate visible endometriotic lesions, without the cure of the disease [79], and majority of drugs are symptomatic, not cytoreductive [80]. Yet it is not known if surgery itself may be incomplete (*i.e.*, microscopic disease) or if other factors, such as aberrant PRs expression of the eutopic endometrium influences recurrence [60] connected to the eutopic endimetrium transcriptome changes compared to non-ill women, indicating abnormalities that predispose to new implants in extrauterine locations after surgical excision of ectopic lesions [81]. Recurrence rate after surgery or medication discontinuation was recorded up to 45% after 5 years [82] and recently one discusses the translation from adjuvant therapy to tertiary endometriosis prevention in postoperative medical care [83]. The moment of medical therapy associated to surgery- before, after, or both before and after surgery is much analyzed, to maximize treatment response, but literature data is still inconclusive [84]. The HT goal is to induce atrophy of endometriotic lesions, even if one missis the ability to predict which medication each individual patient will respond to, being many attempts to find one or more predictive markers [85] to score HT, as it is the immunohistochemical Histo (H) -score on the PRs status, and CYP19A1 expression for the response to progestins, respectively for the need to block estrogen signaling [60]. The high H-score for PRs was proposed to be >80 (associated with 100% positive predictive value), and the low H-score ≤ 5 (associated to 94% negative predictive value), with some authors' comments regarding H-score usage: the score is useful for ectopic endometrium response to progestin- based therapy, not for eutopic endometrium, because the lack of score's correlation to eutopic endometrium. It is recommend to score PRs in the excised ectopic tissues, and to determine the reason for progesterone/progestins/COCs failure. When adhesions/fibrosis are predominant it is sure the non-response to HT, but some PRs expression may indicate an insufficient dosage of progestin or noncompliance with therapy (*i.e.*, inability to tolerate side effects), and for cases with low H-score, patients being PR resistant, it is advised to avoid progestins after surgery in favor of GnRH agonists or GnRH antagonists [86, 87], danazol- rarely used actually, or aromatase inhibitors.

Actual medical therapies allow suppression of endometriotic lesions, women require long term treatment [79] to maintain the benefits, to avoid recurrences, being recognized high rate relapse even after surgery. After surgery one must continue HT with contraceptive pills, or IUD [88] with the aim to preserve ovarian follicles reserve, and because ovarian aging, to try spontaneous pregnancy or ART.

Individual genetic characteristics can affect the bioavailability and pharmacodynamics of HT, mainly estrogen dominance and P4 resistance/attenuance, and, hence, explain part of the variability in the therapeutic response, as it is the polymorphism of CYP3A4/5 involved in levonorgestrel metabolism [89].

One can respond to therapeutic wishes by timing progesterone/progestins administration, and by moving from pure hormonal therapy to drug combination, or to novel molecules capable to restore the various homeostatic disrupted mechamnisms by disease. A number of potential therapeutics are currently in pre-clinical or early clinical studies, fact which may alter further treatment strategies.

4.1 Progesterone/progestins therapy

Kistner [90] was first who postulated that decidualisation observed during pregnancy might cause necrosis, and the consequent elimination of superficial ectopic implants, and this was the logical reasoning for progesterone recommendation, and use to control endometriosis. During pregnancy on assists at ovarian functions suppression, fact that is mimicised by HT in endometriosis [91]. After Kistner RW first initiave in the years 1960, there were used progestins, which are inducing a pseudo-pregnancy endometrial aspect or endometrial atrophy at microscopy [92]. The progestins are synthetic different derivates, such as C-21 progesterone derivates (medroxyprogesterone acetate, MPA, and depot MPA, and dydrogesterone,

(DYD- a semisyntethic progesterone derivate), or C-19 nortestosterone derivates (levonorgestrel, norethisterone, lynestrenol, desogestrel, and dienogest), or the 19-norprogesterone derivates without androgenic activity; nomegestrol acetate – (NOMAC) has a similar anti-gonadotropic activity compared to the 19-nortestosterone derivates with androgenic activity, norethisterone acetate (NETA) [93] and a separate class with drospirenone, the unique progestin [94]. The COCs with the synthetic ethinyl-estradiol (20, 30 μg/pill) plus one of the previously mentioned progestins represent a very important cathegory in the control of eutopic and ectopic endometria from intrinsic abnormal steroids signaling [95]. One must keep in mind the Japanese oppinion [96] that concurrent estrogen action is essential for maximal progestin effect in COC, fact controverted by some studies regarding patients satisfaction on pain alleviation in endometriosis, explained by summerizing endogenous estrogen local levels in ectopic endometrium to that of pills [97] but estrogen priming may be necessary to induce PR in endometriotic lesions [96, 98] as progesterone usually actions on estrogen primed tissue. Progesterone and progestins, alone or in association to a synthetic estrogen are considered first line therapy in endometriosis. The positive response to progestins alone or combined estrogen- progestins may induce only partial improvement, the ectopic sites are not eliminated or some patients do not respond at all [99] being recognized only the quiescence of lesions, at best [100] and when first line therapy fails – in one- third of women because progesterone resistance [79] or it is contraindicated, or it is not tolerated one recommends Gonadotropin-Releasing Hormone (GnRH) agonists, GnRH antagonists, and aromatase inhibitors being used in cases refractory to other therapy. Up to 2021 it was published a single RCT on COCs in endometriosis [101] as Donnez and Dolman [79] mentionned in the last European review. It is described a statistically significant, though modest, improvement in dysmenorrhea with OCPs given for four months compared to *placebo*, and a lack of any beneficial effect of OCPs on non-menstrual pelvic pain and dyspareunia, being appreciated the studies failure to report data on their efficacy according to lesion phenotype [102, 103].

Patients present variable responses to progesterone/progestins, according to their pharmakinetics, to their capacities to reacts to medication (genes, receptors for E2, P4), to metabolize progesterone/progestins connected to their levels of N-Acetyl transferases, associated to drug kinetics control by acetylating and converting active forms into inactive metabolites, to their cytochrome P450 3A (CYP3A) system- one of the most known pathway in steroid hormones metabolism,and P450 3A polymorphism is not precisely known in endometrial patgology [89].

4.1.1 "Old" hormone therapies still active in endometriosis

During the long time of progestins usage it was reported a good rate of patient adherence and satisfaction [104, 105]. There are few direct comparisons between different types of progestins in endometriosis clinical studies, with the scarce evidence suggesting that when given by the same route and the same regimen, the effectiveness may be similar [7]. By binding to PRs, progesterone/the synthetic compounds, administrated orally or by non conventional routes (vaginal [106], intrauterine [107]) induce inhibition of estrogen synthesis through down regulation of ERs [64] and of steroidogenic enzymes in endometrial stromal cells, either by up regulation of the oxidative 17β-HSD type 2, which transforms E2 to E1 [108], being triggered by retinoic acid [109] or by reduction of 17β-HSD type 1 expression, and activity, – as was proved specially for MPA, DYD, dienogest [108, 110] which induces the inhibition of aromatase expression with a low local estrogen production in immortalized human endometrial epithelial cells [111] with inhibition of eutopic and endometriotic cells proliferation, and reducing cells survival by apoptosis induction [112] with limitation of local angiogenesis and neurogenesis (proved with the CD31- a neurovascularisation marker), and linking all these mechanisms, the attenuation of the immune-inflammatory response (proved to be more accentuated on new progestins as drospirenone by its effects on inflammatory cytokines - VEGF, and nerve growth factor) [113] so progesterone/progestins change the morphology of endometrium- ectopic and eutopic with reduction of lesion sizes, but with net differences in their response to these drugs, as experimental and clinical studies demonstrated [7, 114], stages III- IV are not responding. Longitudinal assessment of endometrial morphology has demonstrated that the histology aspects are changing in time: initially one registers secretory differentiation, and after several cycles through ERs down- regulation one registers atrophy with tubular glands, weak secretory vacuolation, and stroma low cellular density [115]. Usually one recommends a HT for long term duration, short term therapy being insufficient to obtain the wanted effects, even with dienogest, – which in a short term therapy demonstrated a high frequency of decidualisation and a tendency of inflammation reduction, but it was not able to induce differences comparable to non- treated cases in terms of necrosis, glandular atrophy and angiogenesis [116] (**Table 1**).

4.1.2 Timing progesterone/progestins for preventing progesterone attenuance and progesterone resistance in endometriosis

The discussion on administration of progesterone from early ages of reproductive period, just to permit P4 to stop endometriosis progression, inflammation, and angiogenesis, by maintainance of ERs, PRs normal ratios in epithelial glands and stroma, is supported by Li et al. study [114] at University of Illinois at Urbana-Champaign, (USA). Endometriosis was induced in two immunocompetent mice groups, differently maintained afterwards: one group with E2, and the second group with E2 and P4 subcutaneously, at every 4 days beginning at 4 days before lesion induction (pre- P4 treatment). The endometriosis-like islands were very quickly developed, with different numbers, aspects and sizes according to steroids administrated- after E2 alone there were yellow, more numerous, larger, with abundant blood vessels and extensive adhesions; after E2 plus P4 were white, smaller, non-vascular, with loose attachment. The microscopy (H&E, special biomarkers, IHC for ER, PR, their genes) have shown marked differences regarding mitotic activity (Ki-67 reduction), glandular secretion, endothelial cells and angiogenesis (CD31 increased when was added P4 before induced endometriosis). Another peculiar aspect in the treated group with E2 plus P4 are the inflammatory response changes - first an increase, and later a reduction of inflammatory cells, and changes of their type in endometriosis-like tissues, with similarities between groups in the first 16 days, and a dramatically changed aspect of inflammation after 24 days from induced endometriosis, such as suppressed production of pro-inflammatory cytokines, and infiltration of immune cells in ectopic sites. The authors debated the P_4 action to alleviate lesion outgrowth and to maintain ERα and PR expression

• P_4 restricts expansion of the ectopic lesions by inhibiting endometrial cell proliferation, and neovascularization
• P_4 suppresses E_2-dependent inflammatory responses in the ectopic lesions
• P4 maintaines ERα/PR-mediated signaling; their loss in the ectopic lesions leads to resistance to P_4 therapy if the treatment is postinduction of lesion

Table 1.
Progesterone alleviates endometriosis, induced in the peritoneal cavities of femele immunecompetent mouse, maintained with estrogen if administered before illness induction (from Li et al. [114]).

when P4 is administrated before lesion induction. The use of RT- qPCR permited the endometrial genes assessment in eutopic and ectopic endometria, showing a progressive down-regulation of miRNA expression corresponding to ESR1, PRs and PR-stromal targets *Hand2* and *Hoxa-10* with time of disease progression, and in contrast a gradually increase of ESR2 miRNA, parallel to increased expression of ESR1, PRs, and *HOXA 10* in ectopic lesions, while *Hand2* expression remained suppressed when P4 was administered before lesion induction (PreP4). The P4 inhibitory effect was not observerd when P4 was started at 4 days after endometriosis induction (Post-P4). The study results clearly indicate that the loss of PR-mediated signaling components is a major causal factor for the P_4 resistance existing in mice with endometriosis. The conclusion is that progesterone supplementation from early moments of disease, when PRs are still present can preserve steroid responsiveness and ameliorate E_2-dependent disease progression, but when at later stage, P4 supplementation has minimum effects, because of PRs absence. The hope is that if PRs women's loss is progressive after disease onset, the add of P4/progestins may action with the wanted effects.

4.1.3 Not all progestins are equal in restoring estrogen- progesterone balance in endometriosis. New trends-dienogest

If there were questions if progestins are all equaly capable of acting on endometriosis lesions to induce apoptosis, or to inhibit cell proliferation, adhesion, invasiveness, angiogenesis/neuroangiogenesis, and inflammation, actually one knows their different actions and effects, according to their biochemical structure, and cross effects on glucocorticoid, mineralocorticoid and androgen receptors [117]. In the last 20 years, starting with the Japanese experiments [118] on rats induced- endometriosis, the progestin dienogest (DNG) was much analyzed in Japon, USA, Europe (The European Clinical Study Program) [119] in order to avoid progesterone resistance or progesterone attenuance, by reducing estrogen deleterious effects on endometrium- normal, eutopic and ectopic increasing PRs expression and decreasing proinflammatory cytokines, and the necessity of "add back" therapy imposed by GhRh agonists [120, 121] as it will be further discussed. It was demonstrated that DNG 2 mg/day (once/day in Europe, and 1 mg twice/day in Japon) [120] after 24–52 weeks of administration reduces lesions size, [122] without changing bleeding pattern [123] and with a good score regarding chronic pelvic pains [120]. Because it was proved an *in vitro* dose-dependent inhibition of human endometrial stomal cells proliferation together with morphological and functional changes [124], an Italian clinical study on 20 cases of endometriosis [125] had evaluated doses of 20 mg/day effects, for 24 weeks, with no comparative study-group, and showed no clinically significant effects on hemostasis, haematologic parameters, thyroid and adrenal, liver functions, glucose and lipid metabolism, or electrolyte balance, with maintainance of mean high-density lipoprotein-3 cholesterol from the baseline.

The morphological studies reported inhibition of endometrial cells proliferation, by down-regulation of ESR2/ESR1 *ratio* [126] and aromatase expression [127] with local estrogen synthesis reduction, and the inhibition of human endometrial stomal cells proliferation, together with functional changes, as it is prolactin synthesis- a typical marker for decidualisation [124] and the association of increased apoptosis in endometriotic lesions [128]. DNG increases the PR-B/PR-A *ratio* in ovarian endometriosis [126] and down-regulates the expression of CYP19A1, and inflammatory, and neuroangiogenesis factors through PR- A and B- isoforms [129]. Some studies have revealed that DNG reverses some alterations of the immune system by increasing natural killer cells in the peritoneal fluid, and spleen, parallel to the decrease of peritoneal fluid cellular content, and lower peritoneal macrophages synthesis of inflammatory cytokine IL-1β [118], and inhibits IL-1β release by the endometriotic epithelial cells [130].

4.1.4 Extended regimen of continuous combined hormonal contraceptives in endometriosis

The continuous regimen or extended cycle vs. cyclic use of combined hormonal contraceptives was first proposed by Loudon [131] in a family planning clinic from Ediburgh (UK) by skipping the tablet-free interval of 7 or 4 days. The innitial proposed non traditional regimen was with 84 active pill with etyhil estradiol 50 μg plus linestrenol 250 μg /day and 7 days free, and it obtained a great adherence in women suffering of endometriosis, according to suppression of withdrawal bleeding, and inducing atrophy in ectopic and eutopic endometrium, as it is recognized by *Cochrane Database Syst Rev*., 2014 [132]. The regimen was recommended with levonorgestrel – LNG (90 or 100 μg/day), drospirenone- DRS (3 mg/day) [133, 134] desogestrel (150 μg/day) [135], NETA (1000 μg/day) [136], and recently dienogest (2 mg/day) [137] as progestins, associated to 20 or 30 μg/day of ethinyl estradiol. The regimen of ethinyl estradiol 20 μg plus LNG 90 μg/day was reported for 364 days at Eastern Virginia Medical School, Norfolk (USA) [138] and in Italy during 6 months with ethinyl estradiol 20 μg plus LNG 100 μg/day [139], or during 3 to 6 months in Germany, Frankfurt University [140, 141], and recently the Italian prospective open label study [137] analyzed ethinyl estradiol 30 μg/day plus dienogest 2 mg/day in a continuous regimen vs. 21/7 to assess quality of life and sexual function in women with endometriosis. The pharmaceutical industry created some drugs combinating ethinyl estradiol 30 μg/LNG 150 mg/day for 84 days plus 7 days *placebo*, or the combination of ethinyl estradiol 30 μg/LNG 150 mg/day for 84 days plus ethinyl estradiol 10 μg/day for 10 days, or of ethinyl estradiol 20 μg/LNG 150 mg/day for 84 days plus ethinyl estradiol 10 μg/day for 10 days [142] after the concept called "tricycle regimen" or "tricycling", first named so in Sweden in 1993 very easy to be followed, and very well appreciated by users [135].

The literature describes some attempts to short free hormones interval for the reduction of hormone withdrawal symptoms, as pelvic pains, headaches [143] and this regimen used LNG, norethindrone (1 mg/day), desogestrel, and norgestimate with ethinyl estradiol 35 μg or less/day. All these attempts were followed by better results of pelvic pain control, but after a longer duration of administration (as after 6 months of norethindrone).

One must consider the tricycle regimen of contraceptives in adolescents suffering of menorrhagia, dysmenorrhea, or with family history of endometriosis, in order to reduce the concerns of a future progress of an eventually later diagnosed endometriosis, existing already findings on this cathegory of women, at the Department of Adolescent Medicine of the University of Pitsburg (USA), with a significant ovarian suppression, endometrial atrophy, no metabolic change, and adolescents safety [144]. At this study one must add a recent one [145] sustaining that women who used the new generation of COC or only progestins have lower circulatory inflammatory biomarkers [IL-6, sTNFR2 (soluble tumor necrosis factor α receptor 2), and in a lower degree C-reactive protein] similar to the effect of a higher number of lifetime ovulatory years. The presence of progesterone after ovulation, the new generation of COCs, and the effects of progestins can be the explanation for the benefits in reducing systemic inflammation; being considered that chronic inflammation reduces ovulation rate in premenopausal women, and ovulation and menstruation increase local inflammation.

There are recent reviews on the comparison of flexible/extended COCs to cyclic COC use in endometriosis, published in 2018 in USA (on dysmenorhheea, non- pelvic pains, dyspareunia [146]), or in Europe [147] and the systematic review (2019) of only 8 RTC published between 1934 and 2018 (of a total 743 studies) on dysmenorrheea [148] and in 2021 [79]. It is shown a statistically significant, though modest, improvement in dysmenorrhea - a reduction of 50% when COCs were given for four months compared to *placebo* [147] and a shorter duration of only 4 days of the pains, with conflicting results on interference with daily activity, pain severity, and pain reccurence [148].

4.1.5 Different routes of administration for progesterone/progestins to increase positive effects in alleviation progesterone attenuation/resistance and estrogen dominance

Since many years one discusses non conventional routes for drug administration in order to avoid the second liver passage, and to increase bioavailable active substance where is necessary. Vaginal route for progesterone and medicated intrauterine devices are most analyzed for their beneficial endometrial effects, without or with less systemic effects of progesterone/progestins.

4.1.5.1 Vaginal route for micronized progesterone

Natural Progesterone has far more anti- inflammatory properties, fewer side effects, is very versatile in how it can be used, and the micronization of P4 is very important, and the oral micronized progesterone capsules were re-directed to be used vaginally [149]. Micronized P4 has a more selective effect on PRs, and results in less interaction with androgenic and mineral-corticoid receptors compared with progestins.

The vaginal route for P4 was proposed since many years ago [150] but the new hypothesis regarding the higher endometrial P4 levels than that obtained after intravenous administration was presented by Cicinelli and de Ziegler [151]. This phenomenon of preferential uterine distribution after vaginal administration was named "first uterine pass effect" [38] or "uterine specificity of vaginal progesterone" [152]. The high uterine level of P4 vaginally administered is explained by various putative modes of transport including direct diffusion through tissue, intracervical aspiration, absorption into the venous or lymphatic circulatory systems and countercurrent vascular exchange with diffusion from utero-vaginal veins/lymphvessels to arteries. While the serum P4 concentration is often low or "subphysiological", endometrial effects show in most cases clear and complete secretory changes, or pseudodecidual aspects, or atrophy after long duration of therapy [153]. In USA at Brigham and Women's Hospital [154] one recommends vaginal gel, cream, or suppositories, in a higher dosage for endometriosis control than that for replacement therapy recommanded in menopause, such as 300 mg twice a day for minimum 3 months, then 300 mg at bed-time.

4.1.5.2 Medicated intrauterine systems to restore estrogen-progesterone balance

The direct application of progesterone or a progestin (usually LNG), or of a SPRM (ulipristal acetate was proposed) was another potential option to control estrogen dominance in eutopic endometrium, for avoidance irregular effects of systemic progestins, considering a consistent inhibition of ERs expression in eutopic endometrium [107, 155] with pain reduction, or to avoid pain relapse in postoperative period, and a total patients' satisfaction when compared to their attention for daily pills intake [156].

4.2 New therapeutic strategies to restore estrogen-progesterone endometrial balance in endometriosis. Selective estrogen receptor modulators (SERMs). Selective progesterone receptor modulators (SPRMs)

Medical literature presents under the name of selective estrogen receptors modulators (SERMs) a relative new cathegory of drugs aimed to target down-regulation of E2 signaling, by a direct binding to ERs in a tissue specific manner [91]. The studies on rat induced endometriosis [157] have shown the reduction of endometriotic lesions by down-regulation of ESR1 and cell proliferation by bazedoxifene or by raloxifene, but in a RCT on administration of raloxifene (180 mg/day) after laparoscopically apparent complete excision of ectopic lesions, it was recorded a shortly time for chronic pain relapse with raloxifene vs. *placebo*, but without recurrence of endometriotic lesions at the second laparoscopy [158] and these results have reduced the enthusiasm for first and second generation of SERMs in endometriosis. The third generation of SERMs administration - basedeoxifene, reduced glands size and number of ectopic sites in mice [159].

The selective progesterone receptor modulators (SPRMs) are known since long time, with the antiprogesterone representative RU 436 or mifepristone. SPRMs were proposed to treat unresponsive cases to progestin treatment, due to progesterone resistance dilemma [160] connected to their direct interaction to progesterone receptors, in order to reduce estrogen- induced cells proliferation and prostaglandins production [161]. Two old multicentres trials on mifepristone showed its efficacy in the endometriosis chronic pain control, with lesions size reduction, although results are mixed [162, 163].

Ulipristal acetate suppressed ectopic endometrium induced in mice, with slow reappearance after discontinuation [100]. After many discussions on the promising evidence of inhibiting human endometrial cell proliferation *in vivo* [164] and on the so-called progesterone receptor modulator-associated endometrial changes (PAEC) recorded after 6 months of therapy, which is reversible after ulipristal discontinuation [164] the liver life threatening complications induced the discontinuation of the study on endometriosis effects [165].

Per global these so called "new" classes of molecules with selective receptors of steroid hormones modulation objectives did not covered the expections in endometriosis, according to women pathologic condition progressively induced on their steroid hormones receptors dysregulation/loss.

4.3 New potential therapeutic perspectives: A combination therapy using agonist of ERβ and the SRC-1 isoform as the next generation of endometriosis therapy to restore estrogen-progesterone signaling balance

Long duration of systemic hypoestrogenism may affect brain, heart, and bones, in young women, and for non responders to first line therapy mentionned above, long term medication with GnRH agonists/ antagonists or aromatase inhibitors cannot be recommended, fact that imposed more researches to try to improve estrogen dominance/progesterone resistance, to stop ectopic tissue growth and disease stage progression with chronic pelvic pains, and infertility. These aims were objectives at the Bayllor College of Medicine, Houston (USA) where it was proposed a combination therapy using an agonist of ER β and the steroid receptor coactivator-1 (SRC 1) isoform as the next generation of endometriosis therapy – Han et al. [44] (**Figure 2**).

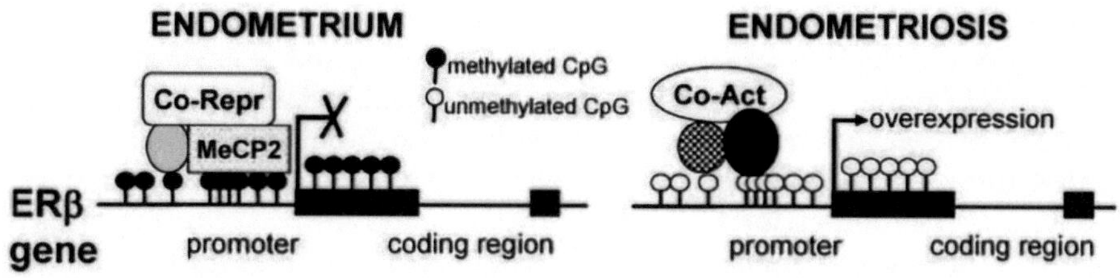

Figure 2.
Hypothesis of Bulun SE, et al. on hypomethylation of ERβ promoter in endometriotic stromal cells vs. hypermethylation, which suppresses the promoter expression in normal endometrium by blocking transcriptional complex including co-activators of ER- β (adapted from Bulun et al. [45]: open acces).

The combination of ERβ- selective agonist and SRC-1 is based on the significant supressive effect of PHTPP on ectopic lesion growth by inhibiting ERβ activity in mice induced endometriosis [166] associated to minimum side effects on ERα, without influences on eutopic endometrium or negative influences on mice fertility. SRC-1 is considered a PR co-activator, and indirectly through it, ERβ may impair PR-mediated signaling in the ectopic lesions, because actually it is no evidence available to show that PR could potentially interact directly with ERβ [167]. These drivers combination allows marked suppression of ectopic lesion growth compared with either individual agents alone, both demonstrating essential roles in early stages of disease pathogenesis [168] specially on apoptosis modulation and inflammation reduction.

4.4 Potential therapeutic options for estrogen dominance control

Several medical treatments for endometriosis directly aim to reduce E2 production or action in order to mitigate E2 dominant conditions, and actually one discusses GhRh agonists, and the new class of GhRh antagonists. These therapies are efficient in cases wishing to conceive, and for the control of chronic pelvic pains- menstrual and non-menstrual [169] but associated hypoestrogenism is cause of many health concerns, requiring hormone "add-back" for long term use [91]. Numerous studies included in the *Cochrane Data Base Systematic Review* (2003) [170] revealed since long time that these effects limit the duration of treatment, which cannot be administered without "add back"/hormone-replacement therapy [171] and treatment cannot be dose-adjusted to alleviate the side effects - Practice Committee of the American Society for Reproductive Medicine (2014) [172].

The recent history of HT for estrogen dominance and progesterone resistance in endometriosis shows that the "old" injectable depot MPA, which can decrease ESR1 and ESR2 while increasing PR-A and PR-B in the eutopic and ectopic endometria [173] has equivalent efficacy to leuprolide- a GnRH agonist, in reducing pain, but with less adverse hypoestrogenic effects on bone density [174].

4.4.1 GnRH agonists. GnRH antagonists

Injectable GnRH agonists (leuprolide, diferelin, nafarelin) are normally second-line treatments. Which decrease hormone levels by down-regulating the pituitary through negative feedback mechanisms [91] and indirectly they favor an endometrial complete silenced hormonal milieu, on the bases of estrogen dominance concept. GnRH agonists have been shown to be effective in reducing endometriosis-related pain [175] with adverse effects – hot flushes, bone mineral density loss, or coronary heart disease, headaches due to a hypoestrogenic state, requiring hormone "add-back" [91]. It was reported a mean percent decrease from baseline in bone mineral density at the lumbar spine of 3.2% at 6 months, and of 6.3% at 12 months after leuprolide alone, and these side effects were associated with rates of discontinuation by 6% because hot flushed, and 8% because of emotional changes [171].

GnRH antagonists, known since long time [176] were in last 10 years under investigation for endometriosis treatment in USA, and Europe according to their capacity to downregulate gonadotropins, without flare-ups like GnRH agonists because they rapidly and directly compete for GnRH receptors [177] and the oral administration is another benefit. Their mechanism of action is different to that of GnRH agonists. After an initial stimulatory phase desensitize GnRH receptors in the pituitary, causing a subsequently depletion of pituitary gonadotropins and full suppression of E2 to levels that are equivalent to those associated with bilateral oophorectomy [178].

Based on Barbieri RL (1992)" estrogen threshold hypothesis" [179] the 2 large multicenters RCTs (Australia, Brazil, Canada, New Zeeland, Poland, USA) [177] have concluded that the new oral Elagolix, a nonpeptide GnRH antagonist, in 2 different doses (one with Elagolix 150 mg/day, and the other RCT with Elagolix 100 mg twice/day) significantly lower scores for dysmenorrhea and non-menstrual pelvic pain than *placebo* after 3 and respectively 6 months of treatment, and dyspareunia at 3 months, with significantly better results in cases on 200 mg/day with respect to the use of rescue analgesic agents at 3 months and 6 months, dyspareunia at 3 months, and rescue opioid use at 3 months less than did those receiving *placebo*. The dysmenorrhea control was better than that of non-menstrual pelvic pains, dysmenorrhea is mostly dependent on cyclic changes in ovarian hormones, whereas the mechanism of non-menstrual pelvic pain are considered more complex [180]. The results allowed the researchers to consider that complete estrogen supression may not be needed to controll endometriosis- associated pain, and estrogen may be adjusted to a level that is adequate to control pain with minimum hypoestrogenic effects (hot flushes, bone mineral density, lipid levels), more frequently claimed in the higher dosage, similar to those induced by GnRH agonists. Elagolix was associated with an antiproliferative effect at each dose, and with endometrial atrophy at higher dose, which was consistent with decreases in endometrial thickness at that dose, but there were considered some limits of the study, as time since endometriosis first surgical diagnosis (in between 10 years), short duration (6 months) of drugs administration. Elagolix did not completely suppress ovulation at either of the two doses [181] being recorded pregnancies, even if patients were recommended to use non – hormonal contraceptive methods during trials. Presently one waits the published results of a phase 3 multicenters RCT in Eastern European countries on an daily oral combination of GnRH antagonist (relugolix) with low doses of estradiol and norethindrone acetate regarding endometrial histology, and endometriosis associated chronic pain, and side effects in comparison to the 4 weeks injectable leuprolide.

4.4.2 Aromatase inhibitors

Aromatase inhibitors (AI), anastrozole and letrozole - the most known derivates, were destinated for control of local E2 levels in many pathologies, and in endometriosis they induce regression of peritoneal lesion size, in a higher degree than MPA [182] by reducing androgen aromatization into estrogens, both in adipose tissue and within endometriotic sites. These drugs are inhibiting endometrial progenitor cells migration to ectopic sites [183], and by increasing apoptosis, and diminishing endometrial VEGF and PGE2 in a mouse model [184] they reduce chronic pelvic pains. AI have significant adverse effects like irregular bleeding, and joint pains [185].

AI action is explained by the promotion of pituitary gonadotropin hormones release, with consequent ovarian stimulation; therefore, they must be combined with a progestin or other method of gonadotropin inhibition to treat endometriosis in premenopausal women [186]. There was compared the association of letrozole (2,5 mg/day) to NETA (2,5 mg/day) vs. NETA (2,5 mg/day) alone, and the Italian open-label study proved a better control for pain and dyspareunia of the drugs association in rectovaginal endometriosis [187] with a better sizes reduction of rectovaginal nodules [188] and of endometrotic ovarian cysts [189]. The effect of the combination of a progestin to an AI is not lasting after termination of HT, so Reis et al. [7] in their published review on progesterone ligands consider letrozole as a second therapeutic- line for selected patients, who fail to respond to first line HT- progesterone/progestins.

5. Potential therapeutic perspectives to restore the estrogen-progesterone receptors balance in endometriosis

The dysregulation of ER and PR in endometrial glandular epithelium and stroma is for sure a pathological mechanism involved in eutopic and ectopic endometrium in women suffering of endometriosis, a disease with onset during embryo-fetal life, and long time duration, sometimes up to death. The prevention and the attemps to maintain or restore the ERα/ERβ, and PR-A/PR-B through their normal genes is one of new potential contemporary therapeutic options.

5.1 Genetic/epigenetic interventions in dysregulated endometrial progesterone responses in endometriosis

Progesterone resistance in endometriosis has genetic causes as PRs gene polymorphisms, altered microRNA expression, and epigenetic changes of PRs and their targets. A consequence of impaired progesterone action is that hormonal therapy is rendered ineffective for a subset of women with endometriosis. Environmental toxins as dioxin may play a role in the genesis of endometriosis by permitting an inflammatory milieu.

5.1.1 Progesterone responsive genes methylation: a cause of a dysregulated progesterone response

The studies at Yale University, New Haven, Connecticut (USA) using RT-qPCR for assessment of endometrial genes in mice induced endometriosis compared to normal mice [190] have demonstrated the silencing or inhibition of P4 target HOX genes (HOXA 10/HOXA 11, known also as genes of receptivity) by promoter hypermethylation - an epigenetic mechanism, which favorizes lack of menstrual cycle variation of PRs distribution, which is proper in normal menstruated women, and this is appreciated as a partial explanation for the refractoriness of some endometriotic lesions to progesterone/progestin therapy [7, 191]. Altered PRs expression or diminished activity may lead to attenuated or dysregulated P4 response in ectopic endometrium, and decreased expression of P4 responsive genes including *HOX genes* in the eutopic endometrium. Cakmak and Taylor [191] and Lee et al. [190] concluded that normal endometrium placed in an ectopic location, in order to create experimental endometriosis led to characteristic changes in gene expression of eutopic endometrium, fact that was previously observed regrading stromal stem cells migration to ectopic sites, without this genetic/epigenetic explanation, and it was controverted. These data were suggestive for the existence of a signal conduction pathway from endometriosis that alters endometrial gene expression through altered *Pgr* signaling and epigenetic programming. The relatively permanent nature of methylation may explain the widespread failure of HT [7]. One discusses about promoters methylation, being controversies if both PRs promoters are methylated, discovering only PR-B methylation, not PR-A [39] or both PRs promoters [192] or DNA methylation of the CG- islands in *PR* promoter, and its gene *HOXA 10* [114] as there are controversions regarding ERs genes (*ESR-1* and *ESR-2*), being hypomethylated CpG island at the *ESR2* promoter region,- involved in primary mechanism responsible for differential expression of *ESR2*, discovered to be increased in ectopic and eutopic endometria [40] while other study from Brazil [192] denies their methylation in eutopic and ectopic endometria.

5.1.2 DNA methylation inhibitor: a new therapeutic perspective/challenge to restore PR-mediated signaling molecules in endometriosis

The women's ectopic and eutopic endometrial progressive loss of PRs and ERα/PR-mediated signaling in the developing ectopic lesions during 7 to 12 years from histologic disease's onset to clinical symptoms/signs permits to health care providers to intervene in the epigenetic regulation therapeutic control.

The animal studies at the University of Illinois at Urbana-Champaign (USA) [114] have shown that a DNA methyltransferase (DNMT) inhibitor, such as Decitabine (DAC, 5-aza-2′-deoxycytidine), an analogue of deoxycytidine that can incorporate into DNA strands and cause DNA demethylation [193] compared to vehicle administration in immunocompetent mice induced endometriosis, treated also with E2 had alleviated lesion growth, and increased expressions of PR protein, and miRNA corresponding to *Esr1*, *Pgr*, *Hand2*, and *Hoxa10*, (P4 target), but not for *Ccl5* and *Ptgs2* in the eutopic endometrium and ectopic sites. The results of the study enable the authors to review the involvement of estrogens and progesterone in eutopic and ectopic endometrium, the epigenetic regulation including DNA methylation, the fact that ERα and ERβ (ESR1 and ESR2), PRs (PRA and B), as well as PR-targets *Hoxa10*, *Gata2/6*, and *Hand2* are susceptible to DNA methyltransferases, leading to an aberrant expression of these molecules in endometriosis.

Early studies showed that the promoter sequences of ERα and ERβ ((ESR1 and ESR2), PRs (PR-A and B), as well as PR-targets *Hoxa10*, *Gata2/6*, and *Hand2* are susceptible to DNA methyl transferases, leading to an aberrant expression of these molecules in endometrial diseases [194] and loss of PR-mediated signaling during disease progression contributes to the increased susceptibility to P_4 resistance in ill women. Li et al. [114] accepted the proposed role of inflammation to provoke widespread changes in the genes and chromatin landscape of lesions, because their analyses showed that DNA methylation in PRs and *Hoxa10* promoters was enhanced in the ectopic lesions in comparison to the normal endometrium, and inhibition of genome-wide DNA methylation in female mice restrained lesion expansion and partially restored target gene expression.

6. Conclusions

Endometriosis is a chronic disease, with possible onset in embryonic life, latency in childhood, reactivation from the menarche, with clinical symptoms and signs difficult to be early accurate assessed during reproductive years. Endometriosis has a progressive evolution, which drives through tissue intrinsic properties to increase lesions size and number, and to functional damages of original eutopic endometrium. The cascade of dysregulations in chromatin machinery is difficult to be stopped by hormone therapy and surgery (associated in different strategies), when the abnormal signaling of steroid hormones has started: endometrial estrogen dominance and progesterone attenuate response up to progesterone resistance, because their genes epigenetic disorders. The 7–12 years delay in diagnosis and proper therapy drives to accentuation of chronic pelvic pains, dyspareunia, dyschezia, infertility/subfertility.

The best therapy is to avoid the dysregulation of steroid hormones signaling, induced initially in ectopic and later in eutopic endometrial stroma and glands, to maintain or to restore the estrogen/progesterone receptors natural balance, which may be possible when an early intervention, from the menarche. One may discuss about timing in starting HT in adolescent girls with family history of endometriosis, precocious dysmenorrheal, menorrhagia, abundant blood and clots loss, favorising menstrual blood reflux.

First line therapy is progesterone/progestins, working in prevention of estrogen dominance and progesterone dysregulated signals, and can maintain their positive effects, when it is early administrated, as animal models have shown. One must recommend this first line therapy, for a long time duration, with a single drug (micronized progesterone, or dienogest, a new progestin) or combined with a synthetic/natural estrogen in COCs, in cyclic or in continuous/extended regimens up to response failure, with the advice to avoid drug discontinuation. Vaginal route for micronized progesterone, IUD with progesterone/levonorgestrel may work better for alleviation of estrogen dominance and progesterone resistance.

GnRH agonists/antagonists- second line therapy, are active in correcting the steroid imbalance, but less than our expectances, even with the new oral molecules (as elagolix), or combination of molecules [GnRH antagonists (relugolix or elagolix) plus an estrogen, or plus an estrogen and a progestin], which were proposed to avoid or to reduce add back therapy. The most recent studied molecule of elagolix may be used no longer than 24 months, because a longer administration may impose add back therapy.

Aromatase inhibitors are also second line therapy, recommended in selected patients for refractory endometriosis, with chronic pelvic pains. Letrozole combination to norethindrone acetate is better than the progestin alone in correcting estrogen dominance, and progesterone resistance.

The new therapeutic perspectives regarding the combination of ER agonists with co-activators, and DNA methylation inhibitors are still in studies at high level technology laboratories, not for current medical use.

Conflict of interest

None.

Author details

Manuela Cristina Russu
Obstetrics and Gynecology, "Dr. I Cantacuzino" Discipline of Obstetrics and Gynecology, "Carol Davila" University of Medicine and Pharmacy, Bucharest, Romania

*Address all correspondence to: manuela_russu@yahoo.com

References

[1] Signorile PG, Baldi F, Bussani R, Baldi A, et al – Embryologic origin of endometriosis: analysis of 101 human female fetuses. J Cell Physiol, 2012; 227 (4):1653- 6; doi: 10.1002/jcp.22888.

[2] Crispi S, Piccolo MT, D'Avino A, Signorile PG, et al – Transcriptional profiling of endometriosis tissues identifies genes related to organogenesis defects Journal of Cellular Physiology: 2013; 226(9): 1927- 1937 DOI: 10.1002/jcp.24358

[3] Brosens I, Gordts S, Benagiano G– Endometriosis in adolescents is a hidden, progressive and severe disease that deserves attention, not just compassion. Hum Reprod.; 2013; 28: 2026-2031.

[4] Secosan C, Balulescu L, Brasoveanu S, Balint O, Pirtea P, Dorin G, et al– Endometriosis in menopause- reniewed attention on a controversial disease Diagnostics (Basel), 2020, 10:134. doi 103390/diagnostics10030134

[5] McKinnon B, Mueller M, Montgomery G– Progesterone resistance in endometriosis: an acquired property? Trends EndocrinolMetab. 2018 Aug;29(8):535-548. doi: 10.1016/j.tem.2018.05.006

[6] Al-Sabbagh M, Lam EW, Brosens JJ– Mechanisms of endometrial progesterone resistance. Mol Cell Endocrinol. 2012; 358: 208-215

[7] Reis MF, Coutinho ML, Vannuccini S, Batteux F, Chapron Ch, Petraglia F – Progesterone receptor ligands for the treatment of endometriosis: the mechanisms behind therapeutic success and failure Human Reproduction Update, July-August 2020, 26 (4) 565-585, https://doi.org/10.1093/humupd/dmaa009

[8] Grümmer R, Traub O, Winterhager E – Gap junction connexin genes cx26 and cx43 are differentially regulated by ovarian steroid hormones in rat endometrium. Endocrinology 1999; 140:2509-2516

[9] Warren LA, Shih A, Renteira SM, Sechkin T, Gregersen PK, et al – Analysis of menstrual effluent: diagnostic potential for endometriosis. Mol Med, 2018; 24 (1), 1; doi: 10.1186/s10020-018-0009-6.

[10] Kondi-Pafiti A, Spanidou-Carvouni H, Papadias K, et al. – Malignant neoplasms arising in endometriosis: clinicopathological study of 14 cases. Clin Exp Obstet Gynecol. 2004;31(4):302-304.

[11] Wheeler JM – Epidemiology of endometriosis-associated infertility. J Reprod Med; 1989*;* 34 41 –46

[12] Giudice LC, Kao LC – Endometriosis. Lancet. 2004;364(9447):1789-1799

[13] Du H, Taylor SH – The Role of *Hox* Genes in Female Reproductive Tract Development, Adult Function, and Fertility. Cold Spring Harb Perspect Med 2015 Nov, 6 (1), a023002. doi: 10.1101/cshperspect.a023002.

[14] Olive DL, Pritts EA – Treatment of endometriosis. *N. Engl J Med;*2001; 345: 266-275.

[15] Giudice LC – Clinical practice. Endometriosis. N Engl J Med. 2010; 362(25):2389-2398

[16] Johnson NP, Hummelshoj L – World Endometriosis Society Montpellier Consortium. Consensus on current management of endometriosis. Hum Reprod 2013*;*28*:*1552-68.

[17] Patel B, Elguero S, Thakore S, Dahoud W, Bedaiwy M, Mesiano S – Role

of nuclear progesterone receptor isoforms in uterine pathophysiology. Hum. Reprod Update. 2015; 21: 155– 73

[18] Tuttlies F, Keckstein J, Ulrich U, Possover M, Tinnerberg HP, et al – ENZIAN-Score, a classification of deep infiltrating endometriosis. 2005, Zentrahl Gynakol, 127(5):275-81

[19] Haas D, Shelb O, Shamiyeh, Oppelt P – The rASRM score and the Enzian classification for endometriosis. Their stengths and weaknesses. Acta Obstet Gynecol. Scand 2012 oct, 92 (1). doi: 10.1111/aogs.12026

[20] Keckstein J, Saridogan E, Ulrich AU, Sillem M, Hudelist G, et al– The ENZIAN classification; A comprehensive non- invasive description system for endometriosis. Acta Obstetricia et Gynecologica Scandinavica, 2021, 100(7), 1165-1175 doi. Org/10.1111/aogs,14099

[21] Starzinski-Powitz A, Zeitvogel A, Schreiner A, Baumann R – In search of pathogenic mechanisms in endometriosis: the challenge for molecular cell biology. Curr Mol Med; 2001; 1 (6): 655-64.

[22] Forte A, Cipollaro M, Galderisi U – Genetic, epigenetic and stem cell alterations in endometriosis: new insights and potential therapeutic perspectives Clin Sci (Lond); 2014; 126(2):123-38. doi: 10.1042/ CS20130099.

[23] Brinton LA, Gridley G, Persson I, Baron J, Bergqvist A– Cancer risk after a hospital discharge diagnosis of endometriosis. Am J Obstet Gynecol. 1997 Mar;176(3):572-9. doi: 10.1016/ s0002-9378(97)70550-7.

[24] Ness RB, Cramer DW, Goodman MT, Wu HA, et al – Infertility, fertility drugs, and ovarian cancer: a pooled analysis of case-control studies. Am J Epidemiol. 2002 Feb 1;155(3):217-24. doi: 10.1093/aje/155.3.217.

[25] Sakr S, Naqvi H, Komm B, Taylor SH– Endometriosis Impairs Bone Marrow-Derived Stem Cell Recruitment to the Uterus Whereas Bazedoxifene Treatment Leads to Endometriosis Regression and Improved Uterine Stem Cell Engraftment. Endocrinology; 2014 Apr; 155(4): 1489-1497

[26] Surrey E, Carter MC, Soliman MA, Khan S, Snabes CM, et al – Patient-completed or symptom-based screening tools for endometriosis: a scoping review. Arch Gynecol Obstet. 2017 Aug; 296 (2):153-165. doi: 10.1007/ s00404-017-4406-9.

[27] Klemmt PA, Carver JG, Koninckx P, Mardon HJ, et al – Endometrial cells from women with endometriosis have increased adhesion and proliferative capacity in response to extracellular matrix components: towards a mechanistic model for endometriosis progression. Hum. Reprod. 2007; 22(12):3139-3147; doi: 10.1210/ jc.2009-0207

[28] Burney OR, Talbi S, Hamilton EA, Chi Vo K, Giudice CL, et al – Gene expression analysis of endometrium reveals progesterone resistance and candidate susceptibility genes in women with endometriosis. Endocrinology. 2007;148:3814-3826; doi:10.1210/ en.2006-1692

[29] Jones JP C, Inuwa MI, Nardo GL, Litta P, Fazleabas TA– Eutopic Endometrium From Women With Endometriosis Shows Altered Ultrastructure and Glycosylation Compared to That From Healthy Controls— A Pilot Observational Study. Reprod. Sci 2009 Jun, 16 (6):559- 572 doi: 10.1177/1933719109332825

[30] Patel BG, Rudnicki M, Yu J, Shu Y, Taylor RN – Progesterone resistance in endometriosis: Origins, consequences and interventions. Acta Obstet. Gynecol. Scand. 2017;96:623-632. doi: 10.1111/aogs.13156

[31] Attia GR, Zeitoun K, Edwards D, Johns A, Carr BR, Bulun SE – Progesterone receptor isoform A but not B is expressed in endometriosis. Journal of Clinical Endocrinology and Metabolism. 2000; 85(8):2897-2902

[32] Burns KA, Rodriguez KF, Hewitt SC, Korach KS, et al– Role of estrogen receptor signaling required for endometriosis-like lesion establishment in a mouse model. Endocrinology. 2012; 153; 3960-3971. doi:10.1210/en.2012-1294

[33] Chrousos GP, MacLusky NJ, Brandon DD, Lipsett MB, et al– Progesterone resistance. Adv Exp Med Biol. 1986;196:317-328. doi: 10.1007/978-1-4684-5101-6_21

[34] Keller DW, Wiest WG, Strckler RC, et al – Pseudocorpus Luteum Insufficiency: A Local Defect of Progesterone Action on Endometrial Stroma. J. Clin. Endocrinol. Metab. 1979:48; (1):127-132

[35] Gellersen B, Brosens IA, Brosens JJ– Decidualization of the human endometrium: mechanisms, functions, and clinical perspectives. Semin Reprod Med; 2007; 25: 445-453

[36] Vasquez YM, DeMayo FJ– Role of nuclear receptors in blastocyst implantation. Semin.Cell.Dev.Biol. 2013;24:724-735.doi: 10.1016/j.semcdb.2013.08.004

[37] Plante BJ, Lessey BA, Taylor RN, Wang W, Bagchi MK, Yuan, et al – G protein-coupled estrogen receptor (GPER) expression in normal and abnormal endometrium. Reprod Sci. 2012; 19(7):684-693. doi: 10.1177/1933719111431000

[38] Groothuis PG, Dassen HH, Romano A– Estrogen and the Endometrium lessons learned from gene expression profilling in rodents and human. Hum Reprod. Update; 2007;13:405-417

[39] Wu Y, Strawn E, Basir Z, Halverson G, Guo SW– Promoter hypermethylation of progesterone receptor isoform B (PR-B) in endometriosis. Epigenetics. 2006;1:106-111. doi: 10.4161/epi.1.2.2766

[40] Xue Q, Lin Z, Cheng YH, Huang CC, Marsh E, Bulun SE, et al – Promoter methylation regulates estrogen receptor 2 in human endometrium and endometriosis. Biol Reprod. 2007;77(4):681-687

[41] Bulun SE, Monsavais D, Pavone ME, Attar E, et al – Role of estrogen receptor-beta in endometriosis. Seminars in reproductive medicine. 2012; 30(1): 39-45.

[42] Hewitt SC, Korach KS– Estrogen Receptors: New Directions in the New Millennium. Endocr. Rev. 2018;39:664-675. doi: 10.1210/er.2018-00087

[43] Mendell JT– MicroRNAs critical regulators of development, cellular physiology and malignancy. Cell Cycle. 2005; 4(9):1179-1184

[44] Han SJ, Jung SY, Wu SP, Hawkins SM, Tsai MJ, et al – Estrogen Receptor beta Modulates Apoptosis Complexes and the Inflammasome to Drive the Pathogenesis of Endometriosis. Cell. 2015;163:960-974. doi: 10.1016/j.cell.2015.10.034

[45] Bulun SE, Cheng YH, Pavone ME, Xue Q, Kim JJ, et al – Estrogen receptor-β, estrogen receptor-α, and progesterone resistance in endometriosis. Semin Reprod Med. 2010;28 (01):036-043; doi: 10.1055/s-0029-1242991

[46] Qi QM, Guo SW, Liu XS – Estrogen biosynthesis and its regulation in endometriosis. Reprod Dev Med. 2017;1(1):55. doi: 10.4103/2096-2924.210698

[47] Simmen RC, Kelley AS – Reversal of fortune: estrogen receptor-β in

endometriosis. J Mol. Endocrinol. 2016; 57(2): F23–F27. doi: 10.1530/JME-16-0080.

[48] Acien P, Velasco I, Gutierrez M, Martinez-Beltran M– Aromatase expression in endometriotic tissues and its relationship to clinical and analytical findings. Fertility and sterility. 2007; 88(1):32-8.

[49] Ferrero S, Remorgida V, Maganza C, Venturini P, et al – Aromatase and endometriosis: estrogens play a role. Annals of the New York Academy of Sciences. 2014; 1317:17-23.

[50] Shafrir AL, Missmer SA – Towards subtypes- deep endometriosis oestrogen receptor α expression Nat. Rev. Endocrinol. 2020 Oct; 16(10):541-542. doi: 10.1038/s41574-020-0394-0

[51] Pluchino N, Mamillapalli R, Wenger J-M, Ramyead L, Taylor SH, et al – Estrogen receptor-α immunoreactivity predicts symptom severity and pain recurrence in deep endometriosis. Fertil Steril,. 2020 Jun;113(6):1224-1231.e1. doi: 10.1016/j.fertnstert.2020.01.036

[52] Dimitriadis E, Stoikos C, Stafford-Bell M, Clark I, Salamonsen LA, et al – Interleukin-11, IL-11 receptor alpha and leukemia inhibitory factor are dysregulated in endometrium of infertile women with endometriosis during the implantation window. J. Reprod. Immunol. 2006; 69:53-64. doi: 10.1016/j.jri.2005.07.004.

[53] Kao LC, Germeyer A, Tulac S, Lobo S, Giudice LC, et al – Expression profiling of endometrium from women with endometriosis reveals candidate genes for disease-based implantation failure and infertility. Endocrinology. 2003;144(7):2870-2881

[54] Osteen KG, Bruner-Tran KL, Eisenberg E – Reduced progesterone action during endometrial maturation: a potential risk factor for the development of endometriosis. Fertil Steril. 2005; 83(3): 529-537.

[55] Arici A, Engin O, Attar E, Olive DL – Modulation of leukemia inhibitory factor gene expression and protein biosynthesis in human endometrium. J. Clin. Endocrinol. Metab. 1995; 80:1908-1915.

[56] Kelleher AM, Behura SK, Burns GW, Young SL, DeMayo FJ, Spencer TE– Integrative analysis of the forkhead box A2 (FOXA2) cistrome for the human endometrium. FASEB J. 2019 Jul; 33(7):8543-8554

[57] Nisolle M, Casanas-Roux F, Wyns C, Donnez J, et al – Immunohistochemical analysis of estrogen and progesterone receptors in endometrium and peritoneal endometriosis: a new quantitative method. *Fertil. Steril.* 1994;62(4):751-759. doi: 10.1016/S0015-0282(16)57000-9.

[58] Shao R, Cao S, Wang X, Feng Y, Billig H – The elusive and controversial roles of estrogen and progesterone receptors in human endometriosis. *Am J Transl Res.* 2014; 6(2):104.

[59] Colón-Caraballo M, García M, Mendoza A, Flores I – Human endometriosis tissue microarray reveals site-specific expression of estrogen receptors, progesterone receptor, and Ki67. *ApplImmunohistochemMolMorphol.* 2019;27(7):491-500. doi: 10.1097/PAI.0000000000000663

[60] Flores VA, Vanhie A, Dang T, Taylor HS – Progesterone receptor status predicts response to progestin therapy in endometriosis. J Clin Endocrinol Metab. 2018;103 (12): 4561-4568. doi: 10.1210/jc.2018-01227.

[61] Nothnick WB – MicroRNAs and Endometriosis: Distinguishing Drivers from Passengers in Disease Pathogenesis.Semin Reprod Med; 2017; 35(2):173-180. doi: 10.1055/s-0037-1599089

[62] McEwan IJ – Nuclear receptors: one big family. Methods in Molecular Biology. 2009; 505 3-18. Doi. org/10.1007/978-1-60327-375-0_1

[63] Mote PA, Balleine RL, McGowan EM, Clarke CL– Heterogeneity of progesterone receptors A and B expression in human endometrial glands and stroma. *Hum Reprod*. 2000 Aug;15Suppl 3:48-56. doi: 10.1093/humrep/15.suppl_3.48.

[64] Brichant G, Nervo P, Albert A, Munaut C, Foidart JM, Nisolle M – Heterogeneity of estrogen receptor α and progesterone receptor distribution in lesions of deep infiltrating endometriosis of untreated women or during exposure to various hormonal treatments. Gynecol Endocrinol. 2018; 34(8):651-655

[65] Lee B, Du H, Taylor HS – Experimental murine endometriosis induces DNA methylation and altered gene expression in eutopic endometrium. *Biol Reprod*. 2009; 80(1):79-85

[66] Han SJ, O'Malley BW – The dynamics of nuclear receptors and nuclear receptor coregulators in the pathogenesis of endometriosis. Hum Reprod Update. 2014 Jul-Aug; 20(4):467-84.

[67] Tranguch S. Smith FD, Dey KS – Progesterone receptor requires a co-chaperone for signalling in uterine biology and implantation. Reprod. Biomed. Online. 2007; 14 (Spec No 1): 39-48

[68] Mishra A, Galvankar M, Singh N, Modi D – Spatial and temporal changes in the expression of steroid hormone receptors in mouse model of endometriosis J. Assist Reprod. Genet, 2020 May;37(5):1069-1081. doi: 10.1007/s10815-020-01725-6

[69] Usadi RS, Lessey BA, Kowalik AI, Meyer WR, Fritz MA– The effects of low luteal phase progesterone concentrations on the histologic and functional characteristics of the endometrium. J. Soc. Gynecol. Investig. 2003; 10 (Suppl 2):386A

[70] Szwarc MM, Lydon JP, O'Malley BW – Steroid receptor coactivators as therapeutic targets in the female reproductive system. J. Steroid Biochem. Mol. Biol. 2015; 154:32-38. doi: 10.1016/j.jsbmb.2015.06.010

[71] Han SJ, Jeong J, Demayo FJ, Xu J, Tsai SY, O'Malley BW, et al – Dynamic cell type specificity of SRC-1 coactivator in modulating uterine progesterone receptor function in mice. Mol. Cell. Biol; 2005;25:8150-8165. doi: 10.1128/MCB.25.18.8150-8165.2005

[72] Kommagani R, Szwarc MM, Kovanci E, Gibbons WE, Lydon JP, et al – Acceleration of the glycolytic flux by steroid receptor coactivator-2 is essential for endometrial decidualization. PLoS Genet. 2013;9:e1003900. doi: 10.1371/journal.pgen.1003900

[73] Mukherjee A, Soyal SM, Fernandez-Valdivia R, Gehin M, O'Malley BW, et al– Steroid receptor coactivator 2 is critical for progesterone-dependent uterine function and mammary morphogenesis in the mouse. Mol. Cell. Biol. 2006;26:6571-6583. doi: 10.1128/MCB.00654-06

[74] Jeong JW, Lee KY, Han SJ, Aronow BJ, Lydon JP, DeMayo FJ et al – The p160 steroid receptor coactivator 2, SRC-2, regulates murine endometrial function and regulates progesterone-independent and -dependent gene expression. Endocrinology. 2007; 148:4238-4250. doi: 10.1210/en.2007-0122

[75] Wykes CB, Clark TJ, Khan KS – Accuracy of laparoscopy in the diagnosis of endometriosis: a systematic quantitative review. *BJOG*. 2004;

111 (11): 1204-1212. doi: 10.1111/j. 1471-0528.2004.00433.x

[76] Hori Y, Committee SG – Diagnostic laparoscopy guidelines : this guideline was prepared by the SAGES guidelines committee and reviewed and approved by the Board of Governors of the society of American gastrointestinal and endoscopic surgeons (SAGES), November 2007. Surg Endosc. 2008;22(5):1353-1383. doi: 10.1007/ s00464-008-9759-5.

[77] Wykes CB, Clark TJ, Chakravati S, et al – Efficacy of laparoscopic excision of visually diagnosed peritoneal endometriosis in the treatment of chronic pelvic pain. *Eur* J Obstet Gynecol Reprod Biol. 2006;125(1): 129-133. doi: 10.1016/j. ejogrb.2005.08.008.

[78] Burney RO, Giudice LC – Pathogenesis and pathophysiology of endometriosis. Fertil Steril. 2012;98(3):511-519. doi: 10.1016/j. fertnstert.2012.06.029.

[79] Donnez J, Dolman M-M – Endometriosis and Medical Therapy: From Progestogens to Progesterone Resistance to GnRH Antagonists: A Review. Journal of Clinical Medicine 2021, 10, 1085. https://doi.org/10.3390/ jcm10051085

[80] Vercellini P, Vigano P, Somigliana E, Fedele L – Endometriosis: pathogenesis and treatment. Nature reviews Endocrinology. 2014;10(5):261-75. doi: 10.1038/nrendo.2013.233

[81] Zhao L, Gu C, Ye M, Han M, et al – Identification of global transcriptome abnormalities and potential biomarkers in eutopic endometria of women with endometriosis: a preliminary study. Biomed Rep. 2017; 6(6):654-662. doi: 10.3892/br.2017.902

[82] Evers J, Dunselman G, Land J, Boucksert F– Is there a solution for recurrent endometriosis? *Br J Clin Pract Suppl* 1991, 72, 45-53

[83] Somigliana E, Vercellini P, Vigano P, Benaglia L, Busnelli A, Fedele L– Postoperative medical therapy after surgical treatment of endometriosis: from adjuvant therapy to tertiary prevention. *J Minim Invasive Gynecol*. 2014;21(3):328-334.

[84] Chen I, Velth V, Choudry AJ, Murji A, Maas J, et al – Pre- and postsurgical medical therapy for endometriosis surgery, 2020 Nov 18;11(11): CD003678. doi: 10.1002/14651858.CD003678.pub3.

[85] Hou Z, Mamillapalli R, Taylor HS– Predictive biomarkers may allow precision therapy of endometriosis. J. Endometr. Pelvic. Pa. 2017; 9:279-285. doi: 10.5301/jeppd.5000311

[86] Vercellini P, Viganò P, Somigliana E, Fedele L– Endometriosis: pathogenesis and treatment. Nat. Rev. Endocrinol. 2014;10(5):261-275.

[87] Taylor HS, Giudice LC, Lessey BA, Abrao MS, Chwalisz K, et al – Treatment of endometriosis-associated pain with elagolix, an oral GnRH antagonist. *N Engl J Med*. 2017; 377(1): 28-40.

[88] Morelli M, Sacchinelli A, Venturella R, Mocciaro R, Zullo F – Postoperative administration of dienogest plus estradiol valerate versus levonorgestrel-releasing intrauterine device for prevention of pain relapse and disease recurrence in endometriosis patients. J. Obstet. Gynaecol. Res. 2013; 39:985-990

[89] Moreno I, Quiñones L, Catalán J, Miranda C, Roco A, Gaete K, et al– Influence of CYP3A4/5 polymorphisms in the pharmacokinetics of levonorgestrel: a pilot study. Biomedica. 2012;32:570-577

[90] Kistner RW – The use of newer progestins in the treatment of

endometriosis.*Am J* Obstet Gynecol 1958: 75 :264-278

[91] Ferrero S, Evangelisti G, Barra F– Current and emerging treatment options for endometriosis. Expert. Opin. Pharmacother. 2018; 19 (10):1109-1125. doi: 10.1080/ 14656566.2018.1494154

[92] Andrews MC, Andrews WC, Strauss AF – Effects of progestin-induced pseudopregnancy on endometriosis: clinical and microscopic studies Am J Obstet Gynecol; 1959; 78: 776-785

[93] Couzinet B, Le Strat N, Brailly S, Schaison G– Comparative effects of cyproterone acetate or a long-acting gonadotropin-releasing hormone agonist in polycystic ovarian disease. J. Clin. Endocrinol. Metab. 1996, 63:1031-1035

[94] Krattenmacher R – Drospirenone: pharmacology and pharmacokinetics of a unique progestogen. Contraception. 2000; 62: 29-38

[95] Gezer A, Oral E – Progestin therapy in endometriosis. *Womens Health (Lond)* 2015;11: 643-652

[96] BonoY, Kyo S, Kiyono T, Mizumoto Y, Fujiwara H, et al – Concurrent estrogen action was essential for maximal progestin effect in oral contraceptives. Fertil Steril 2014; 101; 1337-1343

[97] Casper RF – Progestin-only pills may be a better first-line treatment for endometriosis than combined estrogen-progestin contraceptive pills *Fertil Steril* 2017; 107: 533-536

[98] Vercellini P, Ottolini F, Frattaruolo MP, Buggio L, Somigliana E, et al – Is shifting to a progestin worthwhile when estrogen–progestins are inefficacious for endometriosis-associated pain? Reprod Sci; 2018; 25:674-682

[99] Barra F, Grandi G, Tantari M, Scala C, Ferrero S, et al– A comprehensive review of hormonal and biological therapies for endometriosis: latest developments. Expert. Opin. Biol. Ther. 2019; 19:343-360

[100] Liang B, Wu L, Xu H, Cheung CW, Wang CC, et al – Efficacy, safety and recurrence of new progestins and selective progesterone receptor modulator for the treatment of endometriosis: a comparison study in mice. Reprod. Biol. Endocrinol. 2018, 16: 32

[101] Harada T, Momoeda M, Taketani Y, Hoshiai H, Terakawa N – Low-dose oral contraceptive pill for dysmenorrhea associated with endometriosis: A placebo-controlled, double-blind, randomized trial. Fertil. Steril. 2008, 90, 1583-1588.

[102] Vercellini P, Frattaruolo MP, Buggio L– Toward minimally disruptive management of symptomatic endometriosis: Reducing low-value care and the burden of treatment. Expert Rev. Pharmacoecon. Outcomes Res. 2017, 18, 1-4.

[103] Vercellini P– Are combined hormonal contraceptives the neglected treatment for symptomatic endometriosis? Fertil. Steril. 2018, 110

[104] Andrews WC – Hormone therapy of endometriosis -estrogen, androgens, progestin estrogens. Excerpta Med, 1976; 368:46 –59

[105] Vercellini P, Donati A, Ottolini F, Frassineti A, Somigliana E, et al – A stepped-care approach to symptomatic endometriosis management: a participatory research initiative. Fertil. Steril 2018; 109: 1086-1096

[106] De Lignieres B, Dennerstein L, Backstrom T– Influence of route of administration on progesterone metabolism Maturitas. 1995; 21: 251-257

[107] Engemise SL, Willets JM, Taylor AH, Emembolu JO, Konje JC – Changes in glandular and stromal estrogen and progesterone receptor isoform expression in eutopic and ectopic endometrium following treatment with the levonorgestrel-releasing intrauterine system. Eur. J. Obstet. Gynecol. Reprod. Biol. 2011; 157; 101-106

[108] Beranič N, Rižner TL– Effects of progestins on local estradiol biosynthesis and action in the Z-12 endometriotic epithelial cell line. J. Steroid. Biochem. Mol. Biol. 2012; 132′: 303 – 310

[109] Bulun SE, Yilmaz BD, Sison C, Miyazaki K, Wei J, et al– Endometriosis. Endocr. Rev. 2019; 40, 1048-1079.

[110] Mori T, Ito F, Matsushima H, Takaoka O, Koshiba A, Kitawaki J, et al– Dienogest reduces HSD17β1 expression and activity in endometriosis. *J Endocrinol.* 2015: 225:69-76

[111] Miyashita M, Koga K, Takamura M, Izumi G, Nagai M, Osuga Y, et al – Dienogest reduces proliferation, aromatase expression and angiogenesis, and increases apoptosis in human endometriosis. Gynecol. Endocrinol, 2014: 30: 644-648

[112] Minami T, Kosugi K, Suganuma I, Yamanaka K, Kitawaki J, et al – Antiproliferative and apoptotic effects of norethisterone on endometriotic stromal cells in vitro. Eur. J. Obstet. Gynecol. Reprod. Biol., 2013;166:76-80

[113] Makabe T, Koga K, Miyashita M, Takeuchi A, Sue F, Harada M, et al – Drospirenone reduces inflammatory cytokines, vascular endothelial growth factor (VEGF) and nerve growth factor (NGF) expression in human endometriotic stromal cells. J. Reprod. Immunol. 2017; 119:44-48

[114] Li Y, Adur MK, Kannan A, Davila J, Zhao Y, LI Q, et al – Progesterone Alleviates Endometriosis via Inhibition of Uterine Cell Proliferation, Inflammation and Angiogenesis in an Immunocompetent Mouse Model. PloS One, 2016 Oct 24, 11(10), e0163347, DOI: 10.1371/journal.pone.0163347

[115] Dinh A, Sriprasert I, Williams AR, ArcherDF – A review of the endometrial histologic effects of progestins and progesterone receptor modulators in reproductive age women Contraception 2015; 91:360-367

[116] Mabrouk M, Paradisi R, Arena A, Del Forno S, Seracchioli R, et al – Short-term histopathological effects of dienogest therapy on ovarian endometriomas: in vivo, nonrandomized, controlled trial Gynecol. Endocrinol 2018; 34: 399– 403

[117] Stanczyk FZ, Hapgood JP, Winer S, Mishell DR Jr – Progestogens used in postmenopausal hormone therapy: differences in their pharmacological properties, intracellular actions, and clinical effects. Endocr Rev.2013; 34:171-208

[118] Katsuki Y, Takano Y, Futamura Y, Shibutani Y, Nozawa S, et al – Effects of dienogest, a synthetic steroid, on experimental endometriosis in rats Eur. J. Endocrinol. 1998: 138:216-226

[119] Strowtzki T, Faustmann T, Gerlnger C, Schumacher U, Ahlers C Seitz C – Safety and tolerability of dienogest in endometriosis: Pooled analysis from the European clinical study program. International Journal of Women's Health. 7 (default):393; DOI: 10.2147/WH.S77202

[120] Angioni S, Tinelli R, Colelice V, Socolov R– New trends of progestins treatment of endometriosis Gynecological Endocrinology. August 2014 30(11): 769-773 DOI: 10.3109/09513590.2014.950646

[121] Bedaiwy AM, Allaire C, Afraraj S – Long term medical management of endometriosis with dienogest and with a gonadotropin releasing hormone agonist and add back therapy Fertility and Sterility, 2017, 107, 3, 537-548 doi: 10.1016/j.fertnstert.2016.12.024

[122] Andres M, Alves Lopez L, Baracat Chada E, Podgaec S – Dienogest in the treatment of endometriosis: systematic review. Archives of Gynecology and Obstetrics, March 2015, 292(3); DOI: 10.1007/800404-015-3681-6

[123] Strowitzki T, Faustmann T, Gerlinger C, Seitz C – Dienogest in the treatment of endometriosis-associated pelvic pain: A 12-week, randomized, double-blind, placebo-controlled study. Eur. J. Obstet. Gynecol. Reprod. Biol. 2010;151:193-198. doi: 10.1016/j.ejogrb.2010.04.002

[124] Okada H, Nakajima T, Yoshimura T, Yasuda K, Kanzaki H – The inhibitory effect of dienogest, a synthetic steroid, on the growth of human endometrial stromal cells in vitro. Mol. Hum. Reprod. 2001: 7: 341-347

[125] Artini PG, Volpe A, Angioni S, et al – A comparative randomized study of three different progesterone support of the luteal phase following IVF/ET program. J Endocrinol. Invest 1995; 18:57-62.

[126] Hayashi A, Tanabe A, Kawabe S, Hayashi M, Ohmichi M, et al– Dienogest increases the progesterone receptor isoform B/A ratio in patients with ovarian endometriosis. *J Ovarian Res*2012, 5:31; doi: 10.1186/1757-2215-5-31

[127] Shimizu Y, Mita S, Takeuchi T, Notsu T, Kyo S, et al – Dienogest, a synthetic progestin, inhibits prostaglandin E2 production and aromatase expression by human endometrial epithelial cells in a spheroid culture system. Steroids. 2011;76:60-67. doi: 10.1016/j.steroids.2010.08.010.

[128] Miyashita M, Koga K, Takamura M, Izumi G, Osuga Y, et al – Dienogest reduces proliferation, aromatase expression and angiogenesis, and increases apoptosis in human endometriosis. Gynecol. Endocrinol, 2014: 30: 644-648

[129] Ichioka M, Mita S, Shimizu Y, Imada K, Kyo S,et al – Dienogest, a synthetic progestin, down-regulates expression of CYP19A1 and inflammatory and neuroangiogenesis factors through progesterone receptor isoforms A and B in endometriotic cells. J. Steroid. Biochem. Mol. Biol, 2015;147:103– 110

[130] Mita S, Nakakuki M, Ichioka M, Shimizu Y, Kyo S, er al – Dienogest inhibits C-C motif chemokine ligand 20 expression in human endometriotic epithelial cells. *Eur J* Obstet. Gynecol. Reprod. Biol. 2017; 214:65-–70

[131] Loudon NB – A three month trial of a regimen of oral contraceptives that reduces the frequency of menstruation. Br. Med. J.; 1977 :2: 487-490

[132] Edelman A, Micks E, Gallo MF, Jensen JT, Grimes DA – Continuous or extended cycle vs. cyclic use of combined hormonal contraceptives for contraception. Cochrane Database Syst Rev'2014 Jul 29;7: CD004695. doi: 10.1002/14651858.CD004695.pub3.

[133] Foidart JM, Sulak PJ, Schllschnidt A, et al. The use of an oral contraceptive containing etynyl estradiol and drospirenone in an extended regimen over 136 days. Contraception, 2006; 73: 34-40

[134] Harada T, Kosaka S, Elliesen J, Yasuda M, Momoeda M, et al, – Ethinyl estradiol 20 μg/drospirenone 3 mg in a flexible extended regimen for the management of

endometriosis-associated pelvic pain: a randomized controlled trial. Fertil. Steril 2017; 108:798 –805

[135] Cackrimsnidou AC, Hellberg D, Nillson S, Waldemström U, Sikström B, et al – Long interval treatment regimen with a desogestrel- containing oral contraceptive, Contraception, 1993 sep; 48 (3), 205-16. doi:10.1016/0010-7824 (93)80141-h

[136] Edelman A, Koontz SL, Nichols MD et al – Continuous oral contraceptives. Are bleeding patterns depending on the hormones given ? Obstet. Gynecol; 2006, 1071 657-65

[137] Caruso S, Iraci M, Cianci S, Fava V, Cianci A, et al – Comparative, open-label prospective study on the quality of life and sexual function of women affected by endometriosis-associated pelvic pain on 2mg dienogest/30 µg ethinyl estradiol continuous or 21/7 regimen oral contraceptive. J. Endocrinol. Invest. 2016; 39, 923-931

[138] Archer DF, Jensen JT, Johnson JV, Borisute H, Constantine GD, et al – Evaluation of a continuous regimen of levonorgestrel/ethinyl estradiol: phase 3 study results. Contraception. 74(6):439-45

[139] Benagiano G, Carrara S, Fillippi V– Safety, efficacy and patient satisfaction with continuous daily administration of levonorgestrel/ ethinylestradiol oral contraceptives. Patient Prefer Adherence: 3: 131-43.

[140] Wiegratz J, Kuhl H– Long-cycle treatment with oral contraceptives. Drugs: 64 (21): 2447-62

[141] Kuhl H, Birkhäuser M, Müeck A, Neulen J, Brandle W, et al – Long-cycle treatment in oral contraception. Ther Umsch; 66 (2):101-8. doi: 10.1024/0040-5930.66.2.101

[142] Read MC – New regimens with combined oral contraceptive pills-moving away from traditional contraceptive 21/7 cycle. The European J. of Contraception & Reproductive Health Care, 2010, 12 (suppl 2)

[143] Slak PJ, Scow RG, Preece C, et al – Hormone withdrawal symptoms in oral contraceptives users. Obstetr. Gynecol, 2000, 95: 261-6

[144] Sucato GS, Gerschultz KL – Extended cycle hormonal contraception in adolescents Curr. Opin. Obstet. Gynecol; 2005 Oct;17(5): 461-5.

[145] Huang T, Shafrir LA, Eliasssen A-H, Rexrode KM, Tworoger SS – Estimated Number of Lifetime Ovulatory Years and Its Determinants in Relation to Levels of Circulating Inflammatory Biomarkers. Am. J. Epidemiol; 2020 Jul; 189 (7);660-70 doi: 10.1093/aje/kwz264

[146] Jensen TG, Schiaff W, Gordon K – Use if combined hormonal contraceptives for the treatment of endometriosis related pain: a systematic review of evidence. Fertil Steril 2018 Jul, 110 (1):137-152

[147] Vercellini P, Buggio L, Frattaruolo MP, Borghi A, Somigliana E, et al – Medical treatment of endometriosis-related pain. Best Pract. Res. Clin. Obstet. Gynaecol. 2018; 51:68-91. doi: 10.1016/j. bpobgyn.2018.01.015.

[148] Damm T, Lamvu G, Carrillo J, Ouyang C, Feranec J – Continuous vs cyclic combined hormonal contraceptives for treatment of dysmenorrhea: a systematic review. Contracept X, 2019 Jan; 24:1; 100002

[149] Cicinelli E, de Ziegler D, Alfonso R, Nicoletti R, Bellavia M, Colafiglio G – Endometrial effects, bleeding control, and compliance with a new postmenopausal hormone therapy regimen based on transdermal estradiol

gel, and every-other-day vaginal progesterone in capsules: a 3-year pilot study. Fertil. Steril. 2005; 83: 1859-63.

[150] Price JH, Ismail H, Gorwill RH, Sarda IR – Effect of the suppository base on progesterone delivery from the vagina. Fertil. Steril. 1983, 39,490– 493.

[151] Cicinelli E, de Ziegler D, Alfonso R, Nicoletti R, Bellavia M, Colafiglio G – Endometrial effects, bleeding control, and compliance with a new postmenopausal hormone therapy regimen based on transdermal estradiol gel, and every-other-day vaginal progesterone in capsules: a 3-year pilot study. Fertil. Steril. 2005; 83: 1859-63

[152] Cicinelli1 E, Schonauer LM, Galantino P, Matteo MG, Cassetta R, Pinto V– Mechanisms of uterine specificity of vaginal progesterone. Human Reproduction, 2000; 15, (Suppl. 1), 159-165

[153] Deligdish L – Hormonal ptology of The Endometrium. Modern Pathology 2000, vol 13, 285-294

[154] Davids Landau M, Church K – Should You Opt for Natural Progesterone Treatments for Endometriosis? Brigham and Women's Hospital. website, last updated february 2018

[155] Gomes MKO, Rosa-E-Silva JC, Garcia SB, De Sá Rosa-E-Silva ACJ, Ferriani RA, et al – Effects of the levonorgestrel-releasing intrauterine system on cell proliferation, Fas expression and steroid receptors in endometriosis lesions and normal endometrium *Hum Reprod* 2009;24:2736-2745

[156] Morelli M, SacchinelliA, VenturellaR, MocciaroR, Zullo F – Postoperative administration of dienogest plus estradiol valerate versus levonorgestrel-releasing intrauterine device for prevention of pain relapse and disease recurrence in endometriosis patients. J. Obstet. Gynaecol. Res. 2013; 39:985-990

[157] Yao Z, Shen X, Capodanno I, Donnelly M, Fenyk-Melody J, Vakerich K, et al – Validation of rat endometriosis model by using raloxifene as a positive control for the evaluation of novel SERM compounds. J. Invest. Surg. 2005;18:177-183. doi: 10.1080/08941930591004412.

[158] Stratton P, Sinaii N, Segars J, Koziol D, Nieman LK, et al– Return of chronic pelvic pain from endometriosis after raloxifene treatment: A randomized controlled trial. Obstet. Gynecol. 2008;111:88-96. doi: 10.1097/01.AOG.0000297307.35024.b5.

[159] Kulak J, Jr, Fischer C, Komm B, Taylor HS – Treatment with bazedoxifene, a selective estrogen receptor modulator, causes regression of endometriosis in a mouse model. Endocrinology. 2011;152: 3226-3232. doi: 10.1210/en.2010-1010.

[160] Vercellini P, Cortesi I, Crosignani PG – Progestins for symptomatic endometriosis: A critical analysis of the evidence. Fertil. Steril. 1997;68:393-401. doi: 10.1016/S0015-0282(97)00193-3.

[161] Tosti C, Biscione A, Morgante G, Bifulco G, Luisi S, Petraglia F – Hormonal therapy for endometriosis: From molecular research to bedside. *Eur. J.* Obstet. Gynecol. Reprod. Biol. 2017;209:61-66. doi: 10.1016/j.ejogrb.2016.05.032.

[162] Kettel LM, Murphy AA, Morales AJ, Yen SS – Clinical efficacy of the antiprogesterone RU486 in the treatment of endometriosis and uterine fibroids. Hum. Reprod. 1994;9 (Suppl. 1):116-120. doi: 10.1093/humrep/9.suppl_1.116.

[163] Kettel LM, Murphy AA, Morales AJ, Ulmann A, Baulieu EE,

Yen SS –Treatment of endometriosis with the antiprogesterone mifepristone (RU486) Fertil. Steril. 1996; 65:23-28. doi: 10.1016/S0015-0282(16)58022-4.

[164] Whitaker LH, Murray AA, Matthews R, Shaw G, Critchley HO, et al – Selective progesterone receptor modulator (SPRM) ulipristal acetate (UPA) and its effects on the human endometrium. Hum Reprod 2017; 32:531-543

[165] Fu J, Song H, Zhou M, Zhu H, Wang Y, Chen H, et al – Progesterone receptor modulators for endometriosis. Cochrane Database Syst Rev. 2017;(7)

[166] Compton DR, Sheng S, Carlton KE, Rebacz NA, Katzenellenbogen JA, et al – Pyrazolo[1,5-alpyrimidines] estrogen receptor ligands posssessing estrogen receptor beta antagonist activity. Journal of medicinal chemistry, 2004, 47; 5872-5893

[167] Zheng QM, Mao HL, Zhao YJ, Zhao J, Wei X, Liu PS – Risk of endometrial polyps in women with endometriosis: a meta-analysis. Reproductive biology and endocrinology: 2015;13(1):103. doi: 10.1186/x12958-015-0092-2

[168] Han SJ, Hawkins SM, Begum K, Jung SY, O'Malley BW, et al – A new isoform of steroid receptor coactivator-1 is crucial for pathogenic progression of endometriosis. Nat. Med. 2012;18:1102-1111. doi: 10.1038/nm.2826

[169] Prentice A, Deary AJ, Goldbeck-Wood S, Farquhar C, Smith SK – Gonadotrophin-releasing hormone analogues for pain associated with endometriosis. Cochrane Database Syst Rev 2000: CD000346-CD000346

[170] Sagsveen M, Farmer JE, Prentice A, Breeze A – Gonadotrophin-releasing hormone analogues for endometriosis: bone mineral density. Cochrane Database Syst Rev 2003: CD001297-CD001297

[171] Hornstein MD, Surrey ES, Weisberg GW, Casino LA –Leuprolide acetate depot and hormonal add-back in endometriosis: a 12-month study. Obstet Gynecol 1998; 91: 16-24

[172] Practice Committee of the American Society for Reproductive Medicine –Treatment of pelvic pain associated with endometriosis: a committee opinion. Fertil Steril 2014; 101: 927-935

[173] Sroyraya M, Songkoomkrong S, Changklungmoa N, Poljaroen J, Sobhon P, et al – Differential expressions of estrogen and progesterone receptors in endometria and cyst walls of ovarian endometrioma from women with endometriosis and their responses to depo-medroxyprogesterone acetate treatment. Mol. Cell Probes. 2018; 40:27-36. doi: 10.1016/j.mcp.2018.07.001.

[174] Crosignani PG, Luciano A, Ray A, Bergqvist A – Subcutaneous depot medroxyprogesterone acetate versus leuprolide acetate in the treatment of endometriosis-associated pain. Hum. Reprod. 2006; 21:248-256. doi: 10.1093/humrep/dei290

[175] Brown J, Pan A, Hart RJ – Gonadotrophin-releasing hormone analogues for pain associated with endometriosis. Cochrane Database Syst Rev 2010: CD008475-CD008475

[176] Cetel NS, Rivier J, Vale W, Yen SS – The dynamics of gonadotropin inhibition in women induced by an antagonistic analog of gonadotropin-releasing hormone. J. Clin. Endocrinol. Metab. 1983; 57:62-65. doi: 10.1210/jcem-57-1-62.

[177] Taylor HS, Giudice LC, Lessey BA, Abrao MS, Kotarski J, Watts NB, et al.– Treatment of Endometriosis-Associated Pain with Elagolix, an Oral GnRH Antagonist. N. Engl. J. Med. 2017;

377: 28-40. doi: 10.1056/ NEJMoa1700089.

[178] Maggi R, Cariboni AM, Marelli MM, et al – GnRH and GnRH receptors in the pathophysiology of the human female reproductive system. Hum. Reprod. Update: 2016; 22:358-381

[179] Barbieri RL – Endometriosis and the threshold theory. J Reprod Med, 1992, 43 (3) suppl,287-92

[180] Stratton P, Berkley KJ – Chronic pelvic pain and endometriosis: translational evidence of the relationship and implications. Hum Reprod Update 2011; 17: 327-346

[181] Ng J, Chwalisz K, Carter DC, Klein CE – Dose-dependent suppression of gonadotropins and ovarian hormones by elagolix in healthy premenopausal women. *J* Clin. Endocrinol. Metab. 2017;102:1683-1691

[182] Amsterdam LL, Gentry W, Jobanputra S, Bulun SE – Anastrazole and oral contraceptives: a novel treatment for endometriosis Ferti.l Steril 2005;84:300-304

[183] Ersoy GS, Zolbin MM, Cosar E, Mamillapalli R, Taylor HS– Medical therapies for endometriosis differentially inhibit stem cell recruitment Reprod Sci 2017;24:818-823

[184] Bilotas M, Meresman G, Stella I, Sueldo C, Baranao RI – Effect of aromatase inhibitors on ectopic endometrial growth and peritoneal environment in a mouse model of endometriosis. Fertil. Steril. 2010; 93:2513-2518. doi: 10.1016/j. fertnstert.2009.08.058.

[185] Verma A, Konje JC –Successful treatment of refractory endometriosis-related chronic pelvic pain with aromatase inhibitors in premenopausal patients. Eur. J. Obstet. Gynecol. Reprod. Biol. 2009;143:112-115. doi: 10.1016/j.ejogrb.2008.12.002

[186] Ailawadi RK, Jobanputra S, Kataria M, Gurates B, Bulun SE – Treatment of endometriosis and chronic pelvic pain with letrozole and norethindrone acetate: a pilot study. Fertil. Steril 2004; 81:290-296

[187] Ferrero S, Camerini G, Seracchioli R, Ragni N, Venturini PL, Remorgida V – Letrozole combined with norethisterone acetate compared with norethisterone acetate alone in the treatment of pain symptoms caused by endometriosis. Hum Reprod; 2009; 24: 3033-3041

[188] Ferrero S, Leone Roberti Maggiore U, Scala C, Remorgida V, et al – Changes in the size of rectovaginal endometriotic nodules infiltrating the rectum during hormonal therapies, Arch Gynecol Obstet; 2013;287:447-453

[189] Ferrero S, Remorgida V, Venturini PL, Leone Roberti Maggiore U– Norethisterone acetate versus norethisterone acetate combined with letrozole for the treatment of ovarian endometriotic cysts: a patient preference study Eur. J. Obstet. Gynecol. Reprod. Biol; 2014; 174:117-122

[190] Lee B, Du H, Taylor SH (2009) – Experimental murine endometriosis induces DNA methylation and altered gene expression in eutopic endometrium. Biology of Reproduction, 2009, 80 (1), 79-85

[191] Cakmak H, Taylor HS (2010) – Molecular mechanisms of treatment resistance in endometriosis: the role of progesterone-hox gene interactions. Semin Reprod Med; 2010 28 1 69 74

[192] Meyer J, Zimbardi D, Podgaec S, Amorim RL, Abrao MS, Rainho CA– DNA methylation patterns of steroid receptor genes ESR1, ESR2 and PGR in deep endometriosis compromising the rectum. International journal of molecular medicine. 2014;33(4):897-904. doi:10.3892.ijmm.2014.1637

[193] Slack A, Cervoni N, Pinard M, Szyf M – Feedback regulation of DNA methyltransferase gene expression by methylation. European journal of biochemistry / FEBS. 1999;264(1):191-9

[194] Dyson MT, Roqueiro D, Monsivais D, Ercan CM, Pavone ME, Bulun SE, et al – Genome-wide DNA methylation analysis predicts an epigenetic switch for GATA factor expression in endometriosis. *PLoS Genet.* 2014 Mar; 10(3):e1004158

Chapter 5

The Impact of Endometriosis on Controlled Ovarian Stimulation Outcome

Dragoș Albu and Alice Albu

Abstract

Endometriosis, a frequent condition in reproductive age women, is also associated with infertility by mechanisms incompletely clarified. The effectiveness of endometriosis treatment for infertility is debated, being possible that in vitro fertilization (IVF) offers a better alternative. The response to controlled ovarian stimulation (COS) is an important predictor of live birth, but it might be affected in endometriosis possibly through a decrease of ovarian reserve. Moreover, the predictive value of anti-mullerian hormone (AMH) for the response to COS could be altered by factors disrupting the AMH production in endometriosis. Therefore, we aim to review the literature regarding the response to COS and the AMH production and their predictive value for COS response in patients with endometriosis.

Keywords: endometriosis, controlled ovarian stimulation, in vitro fertilization, oocytes number

1. Introduction

Endometriosis is a frequent disease in reproductive-age women [1], consisting of the presence of endometrial tissue outside the uterine cavity. Endometriosis is frequently associated with infertility, being present in 25–50% of infertile patients [2]. On the other hand, 30–50% of endometriosis patients report difficulties to become pregnant [2]. In a large cohort study, women with endometriosis younger than 35 years old had a two-fold higher risk of infertility in comparison with women without endometriosis [3]. The mechanisms underlying the association between endometriosis and infertility are incompletely clarified, with both anatomical and microenvironmental disturbances being suggested [4]. While in infertile patients with advanced-stage endometriosis anatomical changes might be involved (peritubal and periovarian adhesions), the presence of infertility in milder forms of endometriosis suggests other mechanisms. Thus, decreased ovarian reserve, altered folliculogenesis, oocyte quality and endometrial receptivity were reported as possible contributors to infertility [4].

The extent and severity of endometriosis lesions are variable, ranging from few implants on the pelvic peritoneum to surrounding organs infiltration or extension outside the pelvis. Several grading systems for endometriosis have been created, but their predictive value for fertility is unclear. One of these classification systems, the Endometriosis Fertility Index (EFI) which is based on the scores from the American

Society for Reproductive Medicine (ASRM) system [5] combined with anamnestic and information from surgery, gives a score from 0 to 10 points [6]. It was shown that a score between 0 and 3 is associated with a 10% probability of obtaining pregnancy after 3 years with non-IVF treatments, while a score of 9–10 points is associated with a 75% chance of pregnancy [6, 7]. The predictive value of the EFI score for pregnancy was also confirmed for IVF treatments [8].

The impact of variate treatments for endometriosis on chances to obtain pregnancy and the efficacy of infertility treatments is still a matter of discussion. Thus, whether surgery contributes to the improvement of fertility in endometriosis or is preferable to perform infertility treatments needs further clarification.

In minimal or mild endometriosis without anatomical disruption, it was shown that laparoscopic removal of endometriosis implants improves fertility with an increase of risk ratio of 1.44 [9] and an odds ratio of 1.94 [10]. In a large Canadian multicenter study, the monthly fecundity rate and the 36-week cumulative probability of pregnancy increased from 2.4 to 17.7% for a diagnostic laparoscopy to 4.7 and 30.7% for laparoscopic surgery [11]. However, these rates of pregnancy should be discussed with the patients in the light of similar success rates of 30% after only one cycle of IVF taking into account the age, ovarian reserve or the cost of the treatment [12].

In patients with moderate and severe endometriosis surgery aims to remove large endometriomas and to restore the pelvic anatomy. Data regarding the effect of surgery on fertility in this category of patients are lacking. Excision of endometrioma is controversial in infertile patients taking into account the risk to decrease the ovarian reserve and lack of evidence of benefits on IVF outcome [13].

IVF could be a treatment option for infertility in patients with endometriosis. Therefore, the performance of patients with endometriosis at IVF and their predictors should be clarified to elaborate strategies for ovarian stimulation and to improve IVF outcomes. Oocyte yield at IVF is an important predictor of live birth in the general population of patients performing IVF, but it might be affected by the microenvironmental changes associated with endometriosis. Moreover, the AMH production could be disturbed in endometriosis, possibly interfering with its relationship with the ovarian reserve.

Therefore, the present paper aims to review the literature regarding the association of endometriosis with oocytes number and serum AMH level in infertile patients performing IVF, and the predictive value of AMH for the response to controlled ovarian stimulation.

2. The serum level of AMH in infertile patients with endometriosis

The relationship between endometriosis and serum AMH level is largely debated and data available in infertile women undergoing IVF are scarce. Only a limited number of studies with small study groups evaluated the impact of endometriosis on circulating AMH levels in patients with a wider range of endometriosis lesions [14, 15], most of the studies included only patients with endometrioma. The surgery for endometrioma probably affects the serum AMH level as suggested by two systematic reviews [16, 17] and represents a possible confounder of the relationship between endometrioma and AMH. It was shown that the decrease of serum AMH level after surgery was significant and persistent at 12 months in patients with endometrioma over 7 cm, with bilateral cysts and with endometriosis stage IV [18]. In turn, patients with smaller and unilateral ovarian endometrioma and stage III endometriosis had higher chances to have an only transient decline in circulating AMH [18]. However, a recent meta-analysis showed that the mere presence of endometrioma, without previous surgery, is associated with lower AMH levels in patients without clearly defined fertility status [19]. In this study the serum AMH level was decreased in patients with endometrioma both versus patients with non-endometriotic cysts and with healthy ovaries, suggesting a specific effect of endometriosis independent of mass effect. The dimension of the endometriotic cyst could be an important contributor to the decrease of AMH level, although the available data are limited. In the meta-analysis of Muzii et al. most of the studies included patients with mean endometrioma dimension over 6 cm, being therefore impossible to conclude smaller cysts [19]. A small study found that even endometrioma bigger than 2 cm had lower serum AMH levels in comparison with controls [20]. On the other hand, Yoon et al. failed to find any relationship of ovarian endometrioma size with serum AMH level [21]. A small study with less than 60 patients per study group showed that patients with bilateral endometrioma had lower serum AMH levels in comparison with both unilateral endometrioma and no cysts [22]. Moreover, a negative linear relationship was found between endometrioma size and serum AMH level [22]. A prospective study with 40 women per study group reported that patients with endometrioma have a progressive decline in serum AMH level at an accelerated rate in comparison with patients without endometrioma [23].

Data regarding the impact of a wider range of endometriosis lesions on serum AMH levels are limited. A cross-sectional study that evaluated women surgically explored for a benign gynecological condition irrespective of their fertility status reported a similar serum AMH level in endometriosis patients and controls [24]. Patients in this study presented with various types of endometriosis: endometrioma, deep infiltrating endometriosis and superficial lesions [24]. However, in this study, infertile patients with decreased ovarian reserve might be underrepresented since these patients are more probably referred for reproductive treatments rather than for surgery.

Several studies evaluated the relationship between endometriosis and serum AMH levels in patients with infertility. Thus, Yoo et al. found that infertile patients with endometriosis performing IVF had lower AMH in comparison with male factor infertility patients [14]. In this study, the type of the endometriosis lesions was not specified and the number of patients in the two groups was reduced (43 versus 48). Moreover, patients with and without previous surgery for endometriosis were included, without a significant difference in terms of circulating AMH in these two categories of patients. Ashrafi et al. reported that serum AMH level is decreased in patients with deep infiltrating endometriosis with or without endometrioma and infertility [25]. Another small study showed that infertile patients with endometriosis stage I and II have lower circulating AMH levels in comparison with patients with tubal infertility undergoing IVF [15]. Inal et al. found no difference in serum AMH level in infertile patients with and without endometrioma performing IVF [26]. Shebl et al. studied the serum AMH level in patients undergoing IVF and found a decreased AMH only in patients with endometriosis stage III-IV in comparison with male factor infertility, but not in patients with stage I-II endometriosis [27].

3. The association between endometriosis and oocyte yield in infertile patients performing IVF

The relationship between endometriosis and oocytes yields in infertile patients performing IVF was previously studied, but the results are divergent. Senapati et al. found that patients with endometriosis obtain fewer oocytes in comparison with patients with other causes of infertility undergoing IVF in a big database of

347,185 assisted reproductive technic cycles [28]. In this study, the presence of endometriosis was associated with a lower number of oocytes in patients with isolated endometriosis or association with other causes of infertility, including diminished ovarian reserve [28]. The negative association between endometriosis and oocytes yield was also studied by a meta-analysis that included 20,167 patients with endometriosis and 121,931 without endometriosis [29]. Subgroups with 1703 women with stage III/IV endometriosis were compared with 2227 women with stage I/II endometriosis. Although, a small difference in oocytes yield was observed in favor of non-endometriosis patients, the authors concluded that the quality of the evidence is very low, not allowing meaningful conclusions to be drawn [29]. No significant difference in patients with variate stages of endometriosis was reported [29]. Moreover, in both studies patients with and without previous surgery for endometriosis were included, generating a possible bias [28, 29]. Thus, Dong et al. analyzed only patients with previous surgery for endometriosis and found that patients with stage III/IV endometriosis obtained lower oocytes number in comparison with controls [30], suggesting that surgery for severe endometriosis might negatively affect COS response. Several other studies confirmed the negative association between surgery for endometriosis and oocytes yield in women with advanced-stage endometriosis [31]. In patients operated for endometrioma, laparoscopic cystectomy is associated with decreased oocytes number, with an additional effect of bilateral versus unilateral cystectomy [32]. Similarly, bilateral surgery for endometrioma was shown to decrease the oocytes number in comparison with unoperated patients [33].

Regarding the association of variate types of endometriosis with COS response, a recent meta-analysis found that unoperated endometriomas are associated with reduced oocytes number in IVF cycles [34]. Papaleo et al. found that profound infiltrative endometriosis has an additional negative effect on oocytes yield in comparison with patients with isolated ovarian endometrioma, supporting the hypothesis that variate types of endometriosis lesions can differently impact the ovarian response [35]. In turn, a small study that included only patients with stage I and II endometriosis found similar oocytes number with patients performing IVF for tubal infertility [15].

4. The predictive value of AMH for oocyte yield in endometriosis

Although, circulating AMH levels are considered, in general, a valuable tool for the prediction of the ovarian response to COS, in endometriosis its predictive value might be affected. This hypothesis is supported by studies that demonstrated that AMH production could be influenced independently of the ovarian reserve. However, its predictive value in endometriosis is largely unknown.

Yoo et al. showed that serum AMH level is a significant predictor of oocytes yield in endometriosis patients performing IVF [14], while Wahd et al. found no predictive value of AMH in patients with advanced endometriosis [36]. The lack of the predictive ability of AMH was confirmed in another study that analyzed only patients with endometrioma [26]. The design of the studies and differences in study populations might explain the divergent results of the studies, being possible that more severe endometriosis and endometrioma, especially bigger ones to significantly disrupt the relationship between AMH and ovarian reserve.

Despite the negative relationship between endometriosis and circulating AMH reported by several studies, two reports found an increasing serum AMH level with endometrioma size [37, 38]. If this finding will be confirmed by future studies, a possible explanation is a different impact of endometrioma on AMH production from the other endometriosis lesions. The authors hypothesized that the increasing AMH level could be due to higher discharge in the systemic circulation by increased ovarian blood flow as a consequence of the inflammation and neoangiogenesis found in endometriosis. In support of this hypothesis are the studies that reported increased levels of vascular endothelial growth factor (VEGF) in serum and peritoneal fluid of patients with endometriosis [39]. These increased levels are correlated with microvessels density in the endometriotic tissue [40]. Thus, increased vascularization might contribute to disproportionately higher serum AMH levels in comparison with ovarian reserve, therefore affecting its value as a predictor of COS response in endometriosis. However, this mechanism could be particular to endometrioma as suggested by a study that showed that the gene expression of VEGF is increased only in patients with endometrioma and not in those with deep infiltrating endometriosis [41].

5. The mechanisms explaining the decreased ovarian response and decreased serum AMH level in infertile patients with endometriosis

Besides the mass effect of the endometrioma, other mechanisms might be also involved in the occurrence of reduced oocytes yield since similar oocytes number was found in the contralateral ovary of women with unilateral endometriomas [42]. Moreover, more severe endometriosis seems to have an additional negative impact on oocytes number [35].

Histological studies found that the cortex of ovaries with endometrioma presents decreased follicular density, increased fibrosis, loss of cortex-specific stroma [43] and high density of atretic follicles [44]. Moreover, activated follicular recruitment was observed in ovaries with endometrioma [44], suggesting follicle 'burnout' as a possible cause of decreased follicle number. It was suggested that the structural changes are the consequence of the cytokines produced in the endometriotic tissue which might affect the surrounding ovarian tissue by diffusion [44]. It was also showed that the addition of human endometriotic fluid to mouse preantral follicles decreases the follicles survival rates proportional with the endometriotic fluid supernatant concentration [45]. These data support the hypothesis that endometriotic fluid components can influence the ovarian response to COS through long-term destructive effects of ovarian tissue and, therefore, decreased ovarian reserve, but also by directly influencing the follicles survival [45]. It is also possible that the diffusion of the endometriotic fluid components from the peritoneum or the endometrioma to be able to influence the unaffected ovary function and structure [46].

The decreased serum AMH level in patients with endometriosis might be the consequence of reduced ovarian reserve due to structural ovarian changes. However, it was shown that the endometriotic fluid components can directly induce the dysfunction of the granulosa cells [47]. Tumor necrosis factor (TNF) alpha, one of the cytokines overproduced in endometriosis, was found to be negatively associated with serum AMH level [15], suggesting its involvement in decreased circulating AMH. Indeed, an experimental study showed that TNF alpha administration decreases the expression of AMH in bovine ovarian granulosa cells [48]. In mice, TNF alpha was demonstrated to inhibit the AMH production in testis [49]. Thus, TNF alpha might be the mediator of functional decrease of AMH production in endometriosis.

Another mechanism that can contribute to low oocytes yield is a decreased response to gonadotropin stimulation in endometriosis. Thus, interleukin 1 (IL1) was found to be increased in the peritoneal fluid of patients with endometriosis [50–52]. Il1 is also a regulator of ovarian function, being able to decrease the ovary receptors of FSH and LH [53], thus inducing a reduced sensitivity to gonadotropin stimulation. Moreover, women with endometriosis seem to have a decreased expression of the soluble decoy receptor IL1-RII which can generate an augmentation of IL1 alpha and IL1 beta effects [51, 54].

6. Conclusions

The data available in the literature support a negative association between the presence of an endometrioma and serum AMH level. Moreover, previous surgery for endometrioma is associated with decreased serum AMH level, the risk of the persistence of low AMH being higher in patients with bilateral endometrioma, bigger than 7 cm and with stage IV endometriosis. However, in patients with a wider range of endometriosis without clearly defined fertility status the serum AMH level does not seem to be decreased. In infertile patients with endometriosis available studies suggest lower serum AMH levels, although further research is necessary to clarify this aspect. Moreover, endometriosis seems to negatively impact the oocyte yield, especially in patients with previous surgery for severe endometriosis and endometrioma. The impact of variate types of endometriosis on the oocytes yield is incompletely clarified, the available evidence supporting that endometrioma has a deleterious effect on the ovarian response, with a possible additional negative effect of deep infiltrating endometriosis.

Conflict of interest

The authors declare no conflict of interest.

Author details

Dragoș Albu[1,2] and Alice Albu[2,3]*

1 Reproductive Medicine Department, Medlife Hospital, Bucharest, Romania

2 Carol Davila University of Medicine and Pharmacy, Bucharest, Romania

3 Elias Emergency Hospital Endocrinology and Diabetes Department, Bucharest, Romania

*Address all correspondence to: albualice@yahoo.com

References

[1] Burney RO, Giudice LC. Pathogenesis and pathophysiology of endometriosis. Fertility and Sterility. 2012;**98**(3): 511-519

[2] ASRM. Practice Committee of the American Society for reproductive Medicine Endometriosis and infertility: A committee opinion. Fertility and Sterility. 2012;**98**:591-598

[3] Prescott J, Farland LV, Tobias DK, Gaskins AJ, Spiegelman D, Chavarro JE, et al. A prospective cohort study of endometriosis and subsequent risk of infertility. Human Reproduction. 2016;**31**:1475-1482

[4] Da Broi MG, Ferriani RA, Navarro PA. Ethiopathogenic mechanisms of endometriosis-related infertility. JBRA Assisted Reproduction. 2019;**23**(3):273-280

[5] American Society for Reproductive Medicine. Revised American society for reproductive medicine revised classification of endometriosis. Fertility and Sterility. 1997;**67**:817-821

[6] Adamson GD, Pasta DJ. Endometriosis fertility index: The new, validated endometriosis staging system. Fertility and Sterility. 2010; **94**:1609-1615

[7] Tomassetti C, Geysenbergh B, Meuleman C, Timmerman D, Fieuws S, D'Hooghe T. External validation of the endometriosis fertility index (EFI) staging system for predicting non-ART pregnancy after endometriosis surgery. Human Reproduction. 2013; **28**:1280-1288

[8] Boujenah J, Bonneau C, Hugues JN, Sifer C, Poncelet C. External validation of the endometriosis fertility index in a French population. Fertility and Sterility. 2015;**104**:119-123

[9] Jin X, Ruiz BJ. Laparoscopic surgery for subfertility related to endometriosis: A meta-analysis. Taiwanese Journal of Obstetrics & Gynecology. 2014; **53**:303-308

[10] Duffy JM, Arambage K, Correa FJ, Olive D, Farquhar C, Garry R, et al. Laparoscopic surgery for endometriosis. Cochrane Database of Systematic Reviews. 2014;**4**:CD011031

[11] Marcoux S, Maheux R, Bérubé S. Laparoscopic surgery in infertile women with minimal or mild endometriosis. Canadian Collaborative Group on Endometriosis. The New England Journal of Medicine. 1997;**337**:217-222

[12] Tanbo T, Fedorcsak P. Endometriosis-associated infertility: Aspects of pathophysiological mechanisms and treatment options. Acta Obstetricia et Gynecologica Scandinavica. 2017;**96**:659-667

[13] Benschop L, Farquhar C, van der Poel N, Heineman MJ. Interventions for women with endometrioma prior to assisted reproductive technology. Cochrane Database of Systematic Reviews. 2010;**11**:CD008571

[14] Yoo JH, Cha SH, Park CW, Kim JY, Yang KM, Song IO, et al. Serum anti-Müllerian hormone is a better predictor of ovarian response than FSH and age in IVF patients with endometriosis. Clinical and Experimental Reproductive Medicine. 2011;**38**(4):222-227. DOI: 10.5653/cerm.2011.38.4.222

[15] Falconer H, Sundqvist J, Gemzell-Danielsson K, von Schoultz B, D'Hooghe TM, Fried G. IVF outcome in women with endometriosis in relation to tumour necrosis factor and anti-Müllerian hormone. Reproductive BioMedicine Online. 2009;**18**(4):582-588

[16] Raffi F, Metwally M, Amer S. The impact of excision of ovarian

endometrioma on ovarian reserve: A systematic review and meta-analysis. The Journal of Clinical Endocrinology and Metabolism. 2012;**97**:3146-3154

[17] Somigliana E, Berlanda N, Benaglia L, Viganò P, Vercellini P, Fedele L. Surgical excision of endometriomas and ovarian reserve: A systematic review on serum antimüllerian hormone level modifications. Fertility and Sterility. 2012;**98**:1531-1538

[18] Wang Y, Ruan X, Lu D, Sheng J, Mueck AO. Effect of laparoscopic endometrioma cystectomy on anti-Müllerian hormone (AMH) levels. Gynecological Endocrinology. 2019;**35**(6):494-497

[19] Muzii L, Di Tucci C, Di Feliciantonio M, Galati G, Di Donato V, Musella A, et al. Antimüllerian hormone is reduced in the presence of ovarian endometriomas: A systematic review and meta-analysis. Fertility and Sterility. 2018;**110**(5):932-940.e1. DOI: 10.1016/j.fertnstert.2018.06.025

[20] Uncu G, Kasapoglu I, Ozerkan K, Seyhan A, Yilmaztepe AO, Ata B. Prospective assessment of the impact of endometriomas and their removal on ovarian reserve and determinants of the rate of decline in ovarian reserve. Human Reproduction. 2013;**28**(8):2140-2145. DOI: 10.1093/humrep/det123

[21] Yoon H, Lee H, Kim S, Joo J. The relationship of ovarian endometrioma and its size to the preoperative serum anti-Mullerian hormone level. Ginekologia Polska. 2020;**91**(6):313-319

[22] Karadağ C, Yoldemir T, Karadağ SD, Turgut A. The effects of endometrioma size and bilaterality on ovarian reserve. Journal of Obstetrics and Gynaecology. 2020;**40**(4):531-536. DOI: 10.1080/01443615.2019.1633518

[23] Kasapoglu I, Ata B, Uyaniklar O, Seyhan A, Orhan A, Yildiz Oguz S, et al. Endometrioma-related reduction in ovarian reserve (ERROR): A prospective longitudinal study. Fertility and Sterility. 2018;**110**(1):122-127. DOI: 10.1016/j.fertnstert.2018.03.015

[24] Streuli I, de Ziegler D, Gayet V, Santulli P, Bijaoui G, de Mouzon J, et al. In women with endometriosis anti-Mullerian hormone levels are decreased only in those with previous endometrioma surgery. Human Reproduction. 2012;**27**(11):3294-3303. DOI: 10.1093/humrep/des274

[25] Ashrafi M, Arabipoor A, Hemat M, Salman-Yazdi R. The impact of the localization of endometriosis lesions on ovarian reserve and assisted reproduction techniques outcome. Journal of Obstetrics and Gynaecology. 2019;**39**(1):91-97. DOI: 10.1080/01443615.2018.1465898

[26] Inal ZO, Ustun YE, Yilmaz N, Aktulay A, Bardakci Y, Gulerman C. Does the anti-Müllerian hormone truly reflect ovarian response in women with endometrioma? Journal of Obstetrics and Gynaecology. 2019;**39**(4):516-521

[27] Shebl O, Ebner T, Sommergruber SA, Tews G. Anti muellerian hormone serum levels in women with endometriosis: A case-control study. Gynecological Endocrinology. 2009;**25**(11):713-716. DOI: 10.3109/09513590903159615

[28] Senapati S, Sammel MD, Morse C, Barnhart KT. Impact of endometriosis on in vitro fertilization outcomes: An evaluation of the Society for assisted reproductive technologies database. Fertility and Sterility. 2016;**106**(1):164-171.e1. DOI: 10.1016/j.fertnstert.2016.03.037

[29] MAP B, Teixeira DM, Navarro PAAS, Ferriani RA, Nastri CO, Martins WP. Impact of endometriosis and its staging on assisted reproduction outcome: Systematic review and

meta-analysis. Ultrasound in Obstetrics & Gynecology. 2014;**44**(3):261-278. DOI: 10.1002/uog.13366

[30] Dong X, Liao X, Wang R, Zhang H. The impact of endometriosis on IVF/ICSI outcomes. International Journal of Clinical and Experimental Pathology. 2013;**6**(9):1911-1918

[31] Matalliotakis IM, Cakmak H, Mahutte N, Fragouli Y, Arici A, Sakkas D. Women with advanced-stage endometriosis and previous surgery respond less well to gonadotropin stimulation, but have similar IVF implantation and delivery rates compared with women with tubal factor infertility. Fertility and Sterility. 2007;**88**(6):1568-1572. DOI: 10.1016/j.fertnstert.2007.01.037

[32] Esinler I, Bozdag G, Aybar F, Bayar U, Yarali H. Outcome of in vitro fertilization/intracytoplasmic sperm injection after laparoscopic cystectomy for endometriomas. Fertility and Sterility. 2006;**85**:1730-1735

[33] Somigliana E, Arnoldi M, Benaglia L, Iemmello R, Nicolosi AE, Ragni G. IVF-ICSI outcome in women operated on for bilateral endometriomas. Human Reproduction; **208**(23):1526-1530

[34] Alshehre SM, Narice BF, Fenwick MA, Metwally M. The impact of endometrioma on in vitro fertilisation/intra-cytoplasmic injection IVF/ICSI reproductive outcomes: A systematic review and meta-analysis. Archives of Gynecology and Obstetrics. 2021;**303**(1):3-16. DOI: 10.1007/s00404-020-05796-9

[35] Papaleo E, Ottolina J, Viganò P, Brigante C, Marsiglio E, De Michele F, et al. Deep pelvic endometriosis negatively affects ovarian reserve and the number of oocytes retrieved for in vitro fertilization. Acta Obstetricia et Gynecologica Scandinavica. 2011;**90**(8):878-884. DOI: 10.1111/j.1600-0412.2011.01161.x

[36] Wahd SA, Alalaf SK, Al-Shawaf T, Al-Tawil NG. Ovarian reserve markers and assisted reproductive technique (ART) outcomes in women with advanced endometriosis. Reproductive Biology and Endocrinology. 2014;**12**:120

[37] Marcellin L, Santulli P, Bourdon M, Comte C, Maignien C, Just PA, et al. Serum antimüllerian hormone concentration increases with ovarian endometrioma size. Fertility and Sterility. 2019;**111**(5):5944-5952

[38] Roman H, Chanavaz-Lacheray I, Mircea O, Berby B, Dehan L, Braund S, et al. Large ovarian endometriomas associated with high preoperative anti-Mullerian Hormone levels. RBMOnline. 2021;**42**(1):158-164. DOI: 10.1016/j.rbmo.2020.09.008

[39] McLaren J, Prentice A, Charnock-Jones DS, Smith SK. Vascular endothelial growth factor (VEGF) concentrations are elevated in peritoneal fluid of women with endometriosis. Human Reproduction. 1996;**11**:220-223

[40] Bourlev V, Volkov N, Pavlovitch S, Lets N, Larsson A, Olovsson M. The relationship between microvessel density, proliferative activity and expression of vascular endothelial growth factor-A and its receptors in eutopic endometrium and endometriotic lesions. Reproduction. 2006;**132**:501-509

[41] Filippi I, Carrarelli P, Luisi S, Batteux F, Chapron C, Naldini A, et al. Different expression of hypoxic and angiogenic factors in human endometriotic lesions. Reproductive Sciences. 2016;**23**(4):492-497. DOI: 10.1177/1933719115607978

[42] Yang C, Geng Y, Li Y, Chen C, Gao Y. Impact of ovarian endometrioma on ovarian responsiveness and IVF:

A systematic review and meta-analysis. Reproductive Biomedicine Online. 2015;**31**(1):9-19. DOI: 10.1016/j.rbmo.2015.03.005

[43] Kitajima M, Defrere S, Dolmans MM, Colette S, Squifflet J, Van Langendonckt A, et al. Endometriomas as a possible cause of reduced ovarian reserve in women with endometriosis. Fertility and Sterility. 2011;**96**(3):685-691. DOI: 10.1016/j.fertnstert.2011.06.064

[44] Kitajima M, Dolmans MM, Donnez O, Masuzaki H, Soares M, Donnez J. Enhanced follicular recruitment and atresia in cortex derived from ovaries with endometriomas. Fertility and Sterility. 2014;**101**(4):1031-1037. DOI: 10.1016/j.fertnstert.2013.12.049

[45] Kim SK, Jee BC, Kim SH. Effects of supplementation of human endometriotic fluids on in vitro mouse preantral follicle culture. Reproductive Sciences. 2018;**25**(5):683-689. DOI: 10.1177/1933719116678687

[46] Sanchez AM, Somigliana E, Vercellini P, Pagliardini L, Candiani M, Vigano P. Endometriosis as a detrimental condition for granulosa cell steroidogenesis and development: From molecular alterations to clinical impact. The Journal of Steroid Biochemistry and Molecular Biology. 2016;**155**:35-46

[47] Sanchez AM, Viganò P, Somigliana E, Panina-Bordignon P, Vercellini P, Candiani M. The distinguishing cellular and molecular features of the endometriotic ovarian cyst: From pathophysiology to the potential endometrioma-mediated damage to the ovary. Human Reproduction Update. 2014;**20**(2):217-230. DOI: 10.1093/humupd/dmt053

[48] Glister C, Hatzirodos N, Hummitzsch K, Knight PG, Rodgers RJ. The global effect of follicle-stimulating hormone and tumour necrosis factor α on gene expression in cultured bovine ovarian granulosa cells. BMC Genomics. 2014;**15**:72. DOI: 10.1186/1471-2164-15-72

[49] Hong CY, Park JH, Seo KH, et al. Expression of MIS in the testis is downregulated by tumor necrosis factor alpha through the negative regulation of SF-1 transactivation by NF-kappa B. Molecular Cellular Biology. 2003;**23**:6000-6012

[50] Cheong YC, Shelton JB, Laird SM, Richmond M, Kudesia G, Li TC, et al. IL-1, IL-6 and TNF-alpha concentrations in the peritoneal fluid of women with pelvic adhesions. Human Reproduction. 2002;**17**(1):69-75

[51] Kondera-Anasz Z, Sikora J, Mielczarek-Palacz A, Jońca M. Concentrations of interleukin (IL)-1alpha, IL-1 soluble receptor type II (IL-1 sRII) and IL-1 receptor antagonist (IL-1 Ra) in the peritoneal fluid and serum of infertile women with endometriosis. European Journal of Obstetrics, Gynecology, and Reproductive Biology. 2005;**123**(2):198-203

[52] Sikora J, Mielczarek-Palacz A, Kondera-Anasz Z. Imbalance in cytokines from interleukin-1 family—Role in pathogenesis of endometriosis. American Journal of Reproductive Immunology. 2012;**68**(2):138-145

[53] Brännström M. Potential role of cytokines in ovarian physiology: The case for interleukin-1. In: Leung PCK, Adash EY, editors. The Ovary. 2nd ed. Amsterdam: Elsevier-Academic Press; 2004. pp. 261-271

[54] Kharfi A, Boucher A, Akoum A. Abnormal interleukin-1 receptor type II gene expression in the endometrium of women with endometriosis. Biology of Reproduction. 2002;**66**(2):401-406

Chapter 6

Uterine Embolization as a New Treatment Option in Adenomyosis Uteri

Panagiotis Tsikouras, Fotini Gaitatzi, Stefani Filiou, Spyridon Michalopoulos, Aggeliki Gerede, Tsalikidis Christos, Stefanos Zervoudis, Anastasia Bothou, Xanthi Vatsidou, Anna Chalkidou, Georgios Dragoutsos, Ioannis Tsirkas, Konstantinos Nikolettos, Alexios Alexiou, Irine Babageorgaka, Natalia Sachnova, Nikolaos Panagiotopoulos, Theopi Nalbanti, Panagiotis Simeonidis, Nektaria Kritsotaki, Chrysovalantis Stylianou, Anastasios Vasilopoulos, Sebaidin Perende, Panagiotis Peitsidis, Nikolaos Nikolettos and Vasileios Souftas

Abstract

Adenomyosis is characterized by the development of endometrial ectopic glands and tissue in the myometrium layer in depth greater than 2.5 mm from the endometrial surface of the separative area by -myomas well as by hypertrophy and hyperplasia of the smooth muscles of the myometrium. This is filtration, not mere displacement, of the myometrium, from the endometrium. Clinical symptoms include dysmenorrhea and menorrhagia. It is diffuse (adenomyosis) or focal (adenomyoma), asymmetrically affects the uterine wall of premenopausal women (usually the posterior) and often coexists with myomas. The pathogenesis of adenomyosis remains unknown. The treatment options are: drug therapy, invasive treatment of fibroids: myomectomy (open—intra-abdominal, laparoscopic, hysteroscopic), hysterectomy, myolysis—cryocatalysis, microwave or radiofrequency thermal catalysis (RF-ablation), ultrasound focus catalysis (FUS), laser photocatalysis and percutaneous selective uterine artery embolization (UAE). Embolization remains an alternative and not a substitute of hysterectomy. The medical indication is made on a case-by-case basis, depending on age, desire for pregnancy and the clinical symptoms of adenomyosis.

Keywords: adenomyosis, adenomyoma, uterine artery embolization, conservative therapy, surgical procedures

1. Introduction

Adenomyosis consists of a term that describes the presence of endometrial glands in a layer deep in the myometrium, in a random arrangement and similar histological lesions can be also appeared outside of the uterus, such as the area of the rectal septum [1–3]. Pathogenesis and etiology of adenomyosis development have not been elucidated thoroughly.

Studies in humans and experiments in animals support the hypothesis of endometrial insertion from the myometrium, although the development of adenomyosis from Müller's duct debris at locations outside the uterus is possible from the outset.

The conditions for the development of adenomyosis can be either some "weakness" of the smooth muscle fibers of the myometrium or the increased pressure in the uterine cavity or both. To maintain adenomyosis, relatively high concentrations of estrogen and impaired control of the development of the ectopic endometrium, which is associated with the immune system, may be necessary. Hyperplasia and hypertrophy of smooth muscle fibers are a reflection of the reactive changes in the proliferation of ectopic endometrium. The definitive diagnosis is made after hysterectomy, although efforts have been made to confirm the diagnosis preoperatively with magnetic resonance imaging and endometrial biopsies [4–6].

1.1 Genetic predisposition

Adenomyosis, one of the most common diseases in gynecology with a frequency ranging between 5% and 70%, can significantly affect the quality of life of women with clinical symptoms such as menorrhagia, dysmenorrhea and infertility [7–9]. There are two prevailing theories concerning the origin of adenomyosis. One supports "migration", which concerns the penetration of the endometrium into the myometrium, while the other is based on the metaplastic differentiation of the remaining endometrial stem cells in the myometrium. Mutations that have been observed, almost exclusively, in the KRAS genes, in the presence of adenomyosis, underscore the importance of these genes in the pathogenesis of the disease at the genetic level. This discovery of the cause-effect relationship between the presence of mutations in the aforementioned [7–9]. KRAS genes and adenomyosis refuted the recent theory that the reported molecular abnormalities in adenomyosis are mainly epigenetic or associated with abnormal expression in different genes [7–9]. Most recognized abnormalities regarding gene expression, were associated with excess estrogen formation, progesterone resistance and were related to steroid hormone receptors and other transcription factors. More specifically, mutations have been found, such as the following two P129R, M427I/L429M, which are the most predominant ones, in the ESR1 gene of the estrogen receptor α (ERa) located on chromosome 6q25.1 and appear to be involved in the etiology of adenomyosis [7–9]. It has also been described an association between adenomyosis and deregulation of mechanisms involved in the transition process of epithelial to mesenchymal cells, as occurs in cases of decreased expression of Cadherin-1 (CDH1) protein, as well as in cases of increased Notch I and TGF-β levels [7–9]. Regarding epigenetic factors, it has been suggested that Class I histone deacetylases (HDACs) are involved in promoting gene transcription, as well as DNA methyltransferase (DNMT) proteins involved in DNA methylation are associated with adenomyosis. High levels of HDAC1 and HDAC3 as well as DNMT1 and DNMT3B were found in cases of adenomyosis at the ectopic endometrium. Consequently, epigenetic alterations seem to play an important role in the pathogenesis of adenomyosis, which along with the other aforementioned genetic factors provides knowledge that could potentially lead to advances in the diagnosis and treatment of the disease [7–9].

1.2 History of adenomyosis

In the mid-nineteenth century, Rokitansky described a condition in which elongated endometrial glands were embedded in the hyperplastic endometrial layer. The author mentioned two variants of this condition: the first, in which the glands developed in the muscular wall of the uterus and the second, in which the glands extended to the intrauterine cavity, forming polyps [10]. Several researchers in the 1880s and 1890s considered adenomyosis to be either an embryonic error in the distribution of Müller's ducts or the penetration of the hyperplastic basal endometrium into the myometrium [10–14]. Von Recklinghausen, then argued that adenomyosis is the result of displacement of the mesonephric elements. The researcher reported that these ectopic glands are more commonly found in the posterior wall of the uterus and the area of the cornea, and that these areas consist of remnants of Wolff's pores rather than Müller's ducts [10–14]. Marcus, later described the lymphatic transmission of endometrial elements [14]. Although, this theory has been used to interpret pelvic endometriosis, it also provides a possible explanation for adenomyosis. Marcus, then suggested that there are some miller pluripotent cells in the myometrium, which can differentiate into endometrial cells, offering another possible interpretation for the development of adenomyosis [14]. The cycle is now complete, and most researchers believe that adenomyosis is caused by the penetration of the basic endometrium into the hyperplastic layer of the myometrium. It should be noted that all the organs of the human body, which show cavities, present a sub-orogenic area, except for the uterus. It is believed that the main function of the sub-orogenic region is to inhibit the growth of the glands that line these cavities. The term "uterine adenomyosis" was first used by Frankl in 1925. In 1972 Bird and his colleagues defined adenomyosis as "benign, penetration of the endometrium into the myometrium, which causes diffuse enlargement of the uterus and microscopically presents ectopic, non-neoplastic, endometrial glands and layer, surrounded by hypertrophic and hyperplastic endometrium" [15]. This definition still applies today.

However, it has been described by some researchers as "the presence of endometrial glands and a layer, which are diffuse and deep inside the myometrium". The issue of depth is important as the normal endometrial contribution is usually irregular. Thus, adenomyosis must be distinguished from cases in which there is minimal adhesion of the basal layer of the endometrium surrounded by myometrium and there are two ways to treat it. The first case is the detection of myometrial hypertrophy ("collar around the foci of adenomyosis"), because this type of change is not observed in the intramuscular junction. The second way is to measure the distance between the endomyometrial junction and the nearest adenomyotic site, the size of which must correspond to at least 25% of the total thickness of the myometrium. The second approach is particularly useful in the postmenopausal and pregnant uterus, as in these cases there is generally no muscle hypertrophy around the foci of adenomyosis. Although, many researchers consider adenomyosis as a variety of endometriosis and call it internal endometriosis, adenomyosis should be defined as the presence of endometrial glands and mattresses, located outside the myometrium [10–18].

1.3 Epidemiology

The incidence of adenomyosis varies widely, with rates ranging from 5.7% to 69.6% [19, 20]. Although, some of this discrepancy can be explained by the different histological definitions of adenomyosis, the difference is mainly due to the interest of pathological volumes in making the diagnosis. As a result of the local entity of the condition, the diagnosis of adenomyosis is particularly difficult. In the excellent prospective study by Bird et al. [15], 200 consecutive hysterectomy specimens were examined histologically. When three sections of the myometrium were examined, adenomyosis was found in 62 women (31%). When six more incisions were made, three from the anterior and three from the posterior wall of the uterus, another 61 cases of adenomyosis were diagnosed, increasing the rate from 31 to 61.5% [21–25].

The main reason for the difficulty in determining the true incidence of adenomyosis is mainly due to the fact that published studies report the number of adenomyosis cases, but without mentioning the total number of hysterectomies per age group, so the relative impact of adenomyosis with age has not been defined. Another problem is determining the true frequency is also the fact that in the various studies, only women who undergo a hysterectomy are evaluated, and a selection of cases is applied. In two necropsy studies, the incidence of adenomyosis was reported between 50 and 53.7% [21–25]. Although, these studies had a different choice of cases (excluding women who underwent hysterectomy), they show that the true incidence of adenomyosis is at the highest end of the published frequency range. The woman's interest appears to be related to adenomyosis, as 93% of the women treated had children [21–25]. Although, the numbers tend to mimic the general population, their importance is questionable. If these numbers are real, the observation will confirm an interesting paradox, that is, the number of pregnancies protects against endometriosis, but it is a risk factor for the development of adenomyosis. There does not appear to be a significant association between adenomyosis and another gynecological entity. In a retrospective study of 134 women who underwent a hysterectomy, Vercillini and colleagues found a similar coexistence of adenomyosis with fibroids (23%), with uterine prolapse (19%), with endometrial cancer (28%), with ovarian cancer (28%) and with ovarian cysts (21%) [26].

1.4 Pathogenesis

Although, the exact etiological factors of endometriosis have not been clarified yet, there are many theories on this subject, such as the ones proposed by Ridley [27]. According to the most popular view, adenomyosis is the result of the attachment of the basal layer of the endometrium to the myometrium. In non-uterine areas, the predominant theory concerning the pathogenesis of adenomyosis is the de novo development of ectopic fetal residues of Müller's ducts, since an invasive mechanism of the endometrium into the myometrium has not been established. There are significant differences in the cellular level between the basal layer of the endometrium and the functional layer, such as increased DNA synthesis in the nucleus, and margin formation in the functional layer. In general, the functional layer is considered to be the site of blastocyst implantation while the basal layer provides the possibility of intrauterine regeneration after menstruation. During the period of regeneration of the endometrium, cells from the basal layer glands are in close contact with the endothelial cells having intracellular microfiber/tubular and squamous cell systems [28–30].

These findings support the location of possible migration through amoebic contraction-extension. Such morphological changes have not yet been described in the intrauterine epithelium of adenomyosis. However, in vitro studies have shown that endometrial cells have the penetrating capacity and that their penetration rate is similar to that of cell lines from metastatic bladder carcinoma. This penetrating ability can facilitate the expansion of the basal layer of the endometrium to the myometrium. In MCF-7 cells from breast cancer, tenascin production is stimulated by epidermal growth factors (EGF), which are regulated by hormones. The fact that fibroblasts of the endometrial layer produce tenascine, a fibronectin inhibitor that in turn facilitates the migration of epithelial cells, suggests that there is a complex physicochemical relationship during the growth process of the endometrium in the production phase. Tenascin has been immunohistochemically located around the endometrial glands during the productive phase of the cycle, but not in this position after ovulation [28–30]. Tenascin may mediate the interactions between epithelial and mesenchymal cells, where it inhibits cell adhesion to fibronectin in the endometrial adenomyotic type in the same way as in the normal endometrium.

In a study within situ hybridization and immunohistochemistry, it was found that the endometrial glands in adenomyosis selectively express more human chorionic gonadotropin (hCG) receptor mRNA and immunoreactive receptor protein, compared to the present [31–34]. It seems that HCG/LH receptor expression levels do not differ at different sites of the normal endometrium, but increased expression of this receptor may give epithelial cells the ability to invade the myometrium and form adenomyotic islets. Furthermore, quite interesting is the fact that there is an increased expression of hCG/LH receptors in endometrial carcinomas as well as in non-invasive choriocarcinoma trophoblast cells [31–34]. Studies on steroid hormone receptors in adenomyosis foci have shown dubious results. Thus, some studies reported the absence of progesterone receptors in 40% of adenomyosis cases, while others showed higher concentrations of progesterone receptors than estrogens. Relatively high concentrations of estrogen and progesterone receptors were found in both the basal and adenomyotic endometrium using immunohistochemical detection techniques. Estrogen receptors are a prerequisite for the development of the uterus, which is caused by estrogen [35–38]. Although, there is no clear evidence of a disturbed hormonal environment in most women with adenomyosis, hyperestrogenemia may play a role in the process of endometrial infiltration, as women with adenomyosis have a high rate of endometrial hyperplasia. According to some researchers, a relatively high concentration of estrogen is necessary for the development of both endometriosis and adenomyosis [31–38]. The clinical observation that the destruction of the estrogenic environment with danatrol causes regression of the ectopic endometrium and remission of the associated symptoms of menorrhagia and dysmenorrhea reinforces this hypothesis [31–38]. As in uterine fibroids, estrogen is synthesized and secreted in adenomyotic tissues [31–38]. It was found, therefore, that there is aromatase activity of estrogen sulfatase in the upper part of the myometrium, which contained foci of adenomyosis, by the method of steroid biochemical analysis. The activity of estrogen sulfatase and, in particular, aromatase was higher than that observed in normal adjacent endometrium, leiomyomas and suprauterine endometrium. In addition, endometrial aromatase enzyme activity was inhibited in vitro by up to 50% with the addition of 106 M of danatrol [31–38]. Finally, the presence of aromatase was confirmed in foci of adenomyosis from human matrices by immunohistochemical method and, in particular, in the cytoplasm of glandular epithelial cells, but not in the cytoplasm of stratum cells. The production of estrogen by adenomyotic tissue is further enhanced by the finding of a large number of women with adenomyosis and a high concentration of estradiol (30 pg/ml) in menstrual material compared to those without adenomyosis and normal menstrual cycles [31–38].

Adenomyotic tissue appears to respond well to progesterone with secretory differentiation. Progestogens also enhance aromatase activity in both eutopic endometrium and adenomyotic tissues, thus contributing to the biosynthesis of estrogen in adenomyotic foci.

It is possible, however, that the bioavailability of race steroids alone is not sufficient to develop adenomyosis. It is possible that the myometrium, in cases of adenomyosis, is either predisposed to penetrate the main endometrium, so that benign "penetration" of the endometrium occurs secondarily due to "weak" myometrium, or the morbidity of the uterine scraping, fibromyectomy and cesarean section. Thus, adenomyosis was induced in pregnant rabbits, after scraping one horn of the uterus and fallopian tube, while maintaining the pregnancy in the opposite horn [31–38]. Penetration into the myometrium of the basal layer of the endometrium is enhanced, possibly, by increased intrauterine pressure, which, according to Cullen, can be caused by high circulating progesterone concentrations. The immunohistochemical method has been observed, increased expression of class II antigens of the major histocompatibility complex (HLA-DR) in the glandular cells of the idiopathic endometrium, endometriosis and adenomyosis [31–38]. In addition, the number of macrophages in the myometrium of women with adenomyosis appears to be increased. These macrophages can activate helper T- and B-cells to produce antibodies [31–38]. Phospholipid autoantibodies and significant deposition of immunoglobulins (lgs) or complement factors have been found in women with endometriosis or adenomyosis [31–38]. The exact importance of these immune aberrations in adenomyosis or endometriosis is not currently understood. In vitro experiments have shown that activated CD3+ T cells in the uterus and their secretory product, interferon γ, promote the expression of HLA-DR immunoreactivity in endometrial glandular cells and inhibit their proliferation [31–38]. The closer the endometrial cells are to the activated T cells, the greater the inhibition of their growth. It appears that lymphocyte-like formations, located mainly at the endomyometrial junction, are rich in activated T cells. Their appearance coincides with the maximum suppression of endometrial growth, which is observed both morphologically and with proliferation indices [31–38]. On the contrary, the proliferation of the endometrium is observed, to the greatest extent, near the surface of the endometrium, that is, far enough away from the basal layer, in which these lymphoid formations are found [31–38].

1.5 Pathological anatomy

During a hysterectomy, the adenomyotic uterus is usually spherical or soft. It is swollen in 60% of cases, but rarely exceeds the size of a 12-week pregnant uterus [39]. The uterus weighs from 80 to 200 g. In his classic study, in which a woman's interest determined the weight of the uterus, Langlois reported the upper limit of the normal uterus weight at 130 g for the unmarried woman, at 210 g for the firstborn to the third child, and at 250 g for women with four or more children [40]. With these criteria, excluding cases of fibroids, the weight of the uterus does not increase significantly with adenomyosis. Uterines with adenomyosis are usually hyperemic with thick walls. Although, many researchers have reported that adenomyosis is more common in the posterior wall of the uterus than in the anterior. Bird and colleagues found that the foci of adenomyosis were evenly distributed when receiving six additional incisions for histopathology [15]. These foci may be diffusely dispersed in the myometrium, and may sometimes be large and localized, forming structures called adenomas. The characteristic macroscopic appearance of adenomyosis is due to hypertrophy of the myometrium, which surrounds the endometrium [40–44]. When the entire myometrium, or one of the layers of the uterine wall, is diffusely affected, the uterus increases in size and takes on a spherical shape. During the cross-section of the uterus, the hypertrophic muscular beams are visible, which develop in all directions and surround the foci of adenomyosis. The latter, in some cases, may contain "old" blood with a brown appearance, corresponding to hemolyzed blood and hemosiderin deposits [40–44].

Local infection of the uterus by adenomyosis resembles fibroid. The term adenomyoma is used for the frequent occurrence of adenomyosis. Because the treatment is not neoplastic, the term focal adenomyosis is preferred by Hendrickson and Kempson [40–44]. As adenomyoma is often confused clinically with leiomyoma, which is a benign but neoplastic condition, the term adenoma is accepted. Typically the adenoma does not have clearly defined boundaries because they merge with the normal myometrial environment. In contrast, leiomyomas compress the myometrial environment and have well-defined boundaries [45–50].

Leiomyoma can be nucleated, while adenomyoma can not. Histologically, by the immunohistochemical method, the endometrial glands and the layer in foci of adenomyosis resemble the basal layer of the endometrium. Rarely do they respond to hormonal stimuli, a phenomenon that explains, at least in part, that only in certain cases are hemorrhagic or regenerative morphological findings observed in foci of adenomyosis. The reason for the increased tendency of focal bleeding in deep-seated adenomyotic foci is not understood [45–50]. In contrast, the ectopic endometrium at foci of endometriosis often undergoes circular changes, including degeneration, bleeding, and regeneration, which are similar to those seen in the functional layer of the endometrium. The different frequency of menstrual-type changes may be due to the relatively poor vascularity of the ectopic endometrium, which is a type of primary endometrium, compared to the endometriosis of the endometrium, which is rich in perspiration and is a type of functional layer of the endometrium. However, it appears to retain the ability to proliferate as a result it can develop and be responsible for the failure of amenorrhea or submenorrhea after endometrial destruction operations [45–50]. The secretory changes, which include the degradation of the layer in foci of adenomyosis, are observed mainly during pregnancy and treatment with exogenous progestogens and these changes are made through estrogen and progesterone receptors.

Progesterone effect in the non-pregnant uterus is observed in approximately 30–50% of foci of adenomyosis. During intrauterine pregnancy, 57% of the studies evaluated by Azziz found degeneration [39]. Other authors observed degeneration during pregnancy, only in deep foci, at a depth of at least two low-magnification optical fields, while degeneration was absent or insignificant in foci less than two low-magnification optical fields, the boundary of the basal layer of the endometrium-myometrium [45–52]. It is worth to be mentioned that adenomyosis can often be complicated by hyperplastic disorders up to atypia, while squamous cell carcinoma, mucosal metaplasia, and adenocarcinoma can occur in parallel with adenomyosis.

When the carcinoma is confined to an adenomyotic lesion, it should be considered "intravenous" as the prognosis is no worse than the carcinoma for which the patient underwent surgery. It is not possible to determine histologically whether the adenocarcinomas found in the supracervical uterus in foci of adenomyosis are the primary foci or the expansion of the endometrium into the foci of adenomyotic foci [45–52].

1.6 Clinical symptoms

Approximately 35% of adenomyosis cases are symptomatic [53–56]. In other cases, the most common symptoms are menorrhagia (50%), dysmenorrhea (30%) and uterine bleeding (20%). In some cases, discomfort may be an additional symptom. The frequency and severity of symptoms depend on the extent and depth of adenomyosis [53–56].

The exact cause of menorrhagia in patients with adenomyosis is not known. Menorrhagia may be due to poor contractility of the adenomyotic myometrium and compression of the endometrium by submucosal adenomas or leiomyomas. Mefenamic acid may reduce blood loss, suggesting that prostaglandin F2a (PGF2a) may play a role in the greater blood loss in women with adenomyosis [53–57]. Other factors may include anovulation, hyperplasia and, rarely, endometrial adenocarcinoma. Dysmenorrhea, finally, is due to the irritability of the uterus, which in turn is secondary to the increased amount of blood loss [58–60]. The symptoms associated with adenomyosis have not been analyzed by all researchers. For example, in a study of 136 patients with histologically confirmed adenomyosis, the symptoms were varied, non-specific and, according to the researchers, associated with co-existing pathological conditions such as leiomyomas, endometriosis and polyps, rather than with adenomyosis [58–60]. In another prospective study, there were no differences in the incidence or severity of dysmenorrhea and pelvic pain between 28 women with adenomyosis and 157 controls [58–62]. A study of 23 women with myometrial adenomyosis reported no qualitative differences in spontaneous motility of isolated myometrial tissue during the menstrual cycle, compared with normal uterine fibroids [58–62]. The type of mobility was low-intensity and high-frequency automatic contractions during the reproductive phase, both of which increased during the secretory phase. Histamine-induced contractions of the myometrium were similar to all myometrial tissues tested [58–62].

Because the symptoms of adenomyosis are not specific, it is natural for the disease to be rarely diagnosed preoperatively. Most researchers report a correct preoperative diagnosis in less than 10% of cases [58–62]. However, due to the way the cases are selected, the incomplete pathological examination of the surgical specimens, and the limited number of well-designed studies, the true ability to diagnose adenomyosis is difficult to assess.

1.7 Diagnosis

The clinical diagnosis of adenomyosis is, at best, hypothetical (50%) and more often, it either does not occur (75%) [63–66] or the disease is overdiagnosed (35%) [63–66]. Menorrhagia and dysmenorrhea in a large woman, aged 40–50 years, raise the suspicion, but not the diagnosis, of adenomyosis. The uterus may be diffusely swollen, about the size of a 12-week pregnant uterus, and soft and tender to the touch. In addition, the presence of endometrial hyperplasia at the time of hysterectomy is the only variable directly related to adenomyosis [63–66].

Several researchers have used radiological methods to diagnose adenomyosis. In the largest hysterosalpingography study, Marshak and Eliasoph diagnosed adenomyosis in only 38 of 150 patients with proven adenomyosis [67]. However, they did not report either the total number of patients examined or the frequency of a false-positive diagnosis. The most common findings in hysterosalpingography are endometrial diversions and cellular invasions within the myometrium [67].

This test was considered inaccurate because myometrial adhesions attributed to adenomyosis resemble lymphatic or vascular infiltrations of the pigment. Intra-abdominal ultrasound is not useful in diagnosing adenomyosis. In the late 1970s, a group suggested that abnormal ultrasound areas of the myometrium, 5–7 mm in size, were an ultrasound finding characteristic of generalized adenomyosis [63–66].

This view was subsequently challenged by Siedler et al., who reported generalized uterine enlargement, normal uterine echogenicity, and retention of uterine shape in the majority of women with established adenomyosis. Subsequent studies have failed to clarify this issue [68].

Vaginal ultrasound has been used to diagnose adenomyosis since the early 1990s. Fedele estimated 43 women who would undergo hysterectomy for menorrhagia with preoperative transvaginal ultrasound. He described numerous small subsonic areas of the myometrium, with an abnormal ultrasound outline in 22 women [69].

The sensitivity of the method was estimated at 80% and specialization at 74%. Other researchers reported lower sensitivity, at 48 and 53% [70–80]. Other studies, with a larger number of women, are needed to address this issue [81–85].

Magnetic resonance imaging (MRI) has been applied to pelvic pathology and the initial results in women with adenomyosis are encouraging [75–84]. Mark and his colleagues predicted adenomyosis in eight of 20 women studied with T2 images. Ten of the remaining 12 women were correctly diagnosed with adenomyosis free, while in two the diagnosis was uncertain [70].

The researchers described a typical, wide, low-density area surrounding the normal, high-density, endometrium in women with diffuse adenomyosis. Tiny foci of adenomyosis could not be diagnosed. T2 imaging has a significant advantage over shadowless imaging and that with T1 amplification. MRI has been used to differentially diagnose adenomyosis from leiomyomas [75–85].

Ninety-three patients were evaluated preoperatively and the results were related to surgical pathology. The 16 cases of adenomyosis were diagnosed preoperatively. The wider application of new technology needs, however, further evaluation. In addition, the cost can prevent MRI from becoming a widely used diagnostic test [75–85].

CA-125 is an antigen produced by the ovarian epithelial cells. It is secreted from these cells into the blood and is determined in a variety of gynecological diseases. Some researchers have used the determination of CA-125 levels to predict recurrences of non-mucosal ovarian cancers, while others have used it to diagnose recurrences of endometriosis. In the second case, successive determinations of CA-125 levels [75–85].

was required. In 1985, Takahashi and colleagues reported high preoperative CA-125 levels in six out of seven women with adenomyosis [70]. Although, CA-125 levels were elevated in these women, they were significantly lower than in patients with ovarian cancer. One month after hysterectomy, all women showed normal CA-125 levels. The same researchers, by immunohistochemical method, observed CA-125 production in the glandular epithelium of adenomyosis foci in eight hysterectomy specimens [75–88]. In another study, it was not possible to reproduce these results. In the report of 22 women, 11 of whom had adenomyosis, Halila and colleagues found normal preoperative CA-125 levels in all women with adenomyosis [71, 72]. These levels did not change significantly at one and five weeks after surgery. The cause of the different results in these studies was not clear, but it is hoped that future research will lead to some conclusions [71, 72].

Cysteine and leucine aminopeptidase levels have been used as possible markers of adenomyosis. Levels of these enzymes are elevated in various benign and malignant conditions of the uterus and ovaries [75–88].

However, no control studies have been performed to evaluate the clinical utility of these measurements. Although, adenomyosis can be diagnosed after a needle biopsy of the uterus, the sensitivity of this method is low and depends on the number of biopsies and the depth of penetration of the adenomyosis. This technique is of little or no importance in the diagnosis of minimal or moderate disease, but can provide histological confirmation in cases with extensive myometrial infiltration. If the biopsy confirms the diagnosis, women should be identified based on their history and tested for transvaginal ultrasound and MRI. These diagnostic methods can also help determine the location of the biopsy. However, myometrial biopsy, as a routine method, in women with pelvic pain should not be performed [75–88].

1.8 Treatment

Hysterectomy surgery remains the key approach in both the diagnosis and treatment of adenomyosis until a safer and more effective method of immediate biopsy is found. The only way to accurately diagnose adenomyosis is to remove the uterus, which also provides treatment for this condition, whereas prolactin, progesterone and growth hormone appear to accelerate the development of the disease [89–94].

RU 486, an anti-progesterone agent that inhibits the action of progesterone on its receptors in the uterus, suppresses the development of adenomyosis if administered for 30 days. Of course, they also require studies in humans [89–94]. There is evidence that progesterone promotes the development of adenomyosis in humans as well as in muscles [89–94]. Danazol, an antigonadotropic derivative of testosterone 17α-ethinyl, has not been widely used in the treatment of adenomyosis [88].

From June 1993 to August 2000, Tamaoaka et al. treated adenomyosis women with endometrial glomeruli containing danatrol, and observed a marked reduction in dysmenorrhea and levels of CA-125 in women with endometrial hyperplasia. The histopathological findings of hyperplasia disappeared during the use of these endometrial glomeruli. The mechanism of the direct action of danatrol in endometrial hyperplasia has not been fully elucidated [89–94].

Hormone therapy with progestogens or gonadotropin-releasing hypothalamic hormone analogs (GnRH-α) could be as effective as in endometriosis [94–96]. However, an increase in uterine size and a recurrence of symptoms occur within six months of stopping treatment. Conservative surgical treatment may be helpful in some patients, although follow-up of women after such surgery is limited to three years [96–98].

The activity of one orally administered metalloproteinase inhibitor (ONO-4817) in the development of adenomyosis was recently tested experimentally by anterior pituitary gland transplantation into muscle. The results indicate that this drug could be activated the development of adenomyosis [96–98].

2. Uterine artery embolization

The uterine artery embolization (UAE) has been used successfully for refractory gynecologic problems in premenopausal women like: hemorrhage, pain, bulk symptoms, or a combination of them despite previously performed surgical procedures (myomectomy, adenomectomy) or medical treatment. The desire for minimally invasive alternatives for the management of symptomatic adenomyosis premenopausal women prompts interventional radiologists to propose UAE as an alternative treatment to surgical treatment of adenomyosis. According to various reports, the ability to improve menstrual disorders and symptoms of premenopausal women through UAE without the need for surgical procedures led to this method becoming famous. However, despite the positive comments of several reports exist no prospective randomized trials to determine the relative safety effectiveness of UAE compared either to surgical or medical options [78–84]. The cooperation between a gynecologist and interventional radiologist is obligatory to establish optimal clinical guidelines for premenopausal women care due to preinterventional consultation, procedural course and postprocedural follow up require gynecological and also radiological services.

2.1 UAE technical procedure

The target of the UAE is to administrate material polyvinyl alcohol (PVA). Microspheres or gelatin-coated tris-acryl polymer microspheres bilateral in uterine arteries to interrupt or reduce the blood supply at the level of the arterioles and to produce irretrievable ischemic damage, degeneration and shrinkage of adenomyosis focus without causing permanent damage to uterus. The target of UAE is an interruption or reduction of the blood supply of fibroids at the level of the arterioles after bilateral (from left and right) super-selective catheterization with microcatheters of the arteries that supply the fibroids and injection of acryl polymer embolospheres with a diameter of 500–900 μm for provocation of irretrievable ischemic damage to the fibroids. The aspects of the technical approach of UAE are summarized and described as follows: A single right femoral artery is typically catheterized after intravenous local analgesia and after that is performed pelvic arteriography to define the vascular tree and identifiy both uterine arteries. All UAE procedures were carried out in the angio suite with a digital subtraction angiography (DSA) system. Except this is of great importance to exclude present vascular abnormalities. The goal of UAE is partial or complete occlusion of both uterine arteries branches which led to adenomyosis focus with polyvinyl alcohol (PVA). Microspheres or gelatin-coated tris-acryl polymer microspheres and after the embolization of the above-mentioned vessels may produce effective infraction of adenomyosis focus associated due to moderate or severe pain. It is very important to sparing of cervical and vaginal branches, vasoconstriction avoidance, catheter 4-F retraction in the internal iliac artery, after the microcatheter placement.

Caution for anatomic variances:

atypical origin of uterine arteries, ovarian/uterine tube arteries deriving from uterine arteries, multiple arteries branching instead of one artery, absence of uterine arteries, origin from ovarian arteries or round ligament arteries, avoidance of embolization of the ascending branches to the ovary and descending branches to the cervix and the vagina.

After the selective catheterization of the uterine artery visualization with contras, if major ovary branch is visualized micro catheter is moved superelectively inside the ovary branch and the embolization of the supply to the ovary is done first with microspheres or big embolospheres with a diameter 900 μm. Technical difficulties include severe cannulating of arteries due to anatomic variations, arterial spasm, recently use of gonadotropin releasing hormone agonist, uterine perfusion from collateral ovarian vasculature. During the procedure, analgesic treatment (paracetamol and morphine) is administered wherever it is necessary.

3. Our experience with UAE treatment in adenomyosis premenopausal women

Between April 2008 and 2021 sixty-four premenopausal women from our department Obstetrics and Gynecology, with symptomatic adenomyosis (diffuse adenomyosis), focal (adenomyoma) or coexisting with uterine myomas in fourty cases, ten cases and fourteen cases respectively underwent uterine artery embolization (UAE) in cooperation with Interventional Radiology department of Democritus University of Thrace, Greece. All procedures were performed by the institutional ethical standards and with the 1964 Helsinki Declaration.

Informed consent was obtained from all individual participants included in the study. All study participants with adenomyosis with or without concomitant fibroids were assessed for treatment by an experienced gynecologist.

With a medical history, the main symptoms were divided into the following categories: menstrual bleeding, pelvic pain (rated on a VAS score from 0 to 10, with 0 representing no pain and 10 unbearable pain), urinary discomfort, bleeding pain, massive symptoms, combination despite previous treatment, and health-related quality of life effects (restrictions on daily activities, energy/mood, self-awareness, and sexual function). Each participant then underwent a gynecological clinical examination, also transvaginal ultrasound followed by an MRI study. All imaging findings [US/MRI transvaginal ultrasound in either a Tesla 1 scanner (GE Healthcare) or a 1.5 Tesla magnet (Philips Multiva)] were then evaluated by an experienced gynecologist and invasive radiologist for possible treatment in the UAE. We present from our study participants Figures from a case with mixed adenomyosis and myoma uteri (**Figures 1–6**). Additional laboratory tests were performed that included platelet count, clotting time, and renal function markers (creatinine and glomerular filtration rate). All the methods and procedures followed in the present study obey the basic ethical rules. The study was

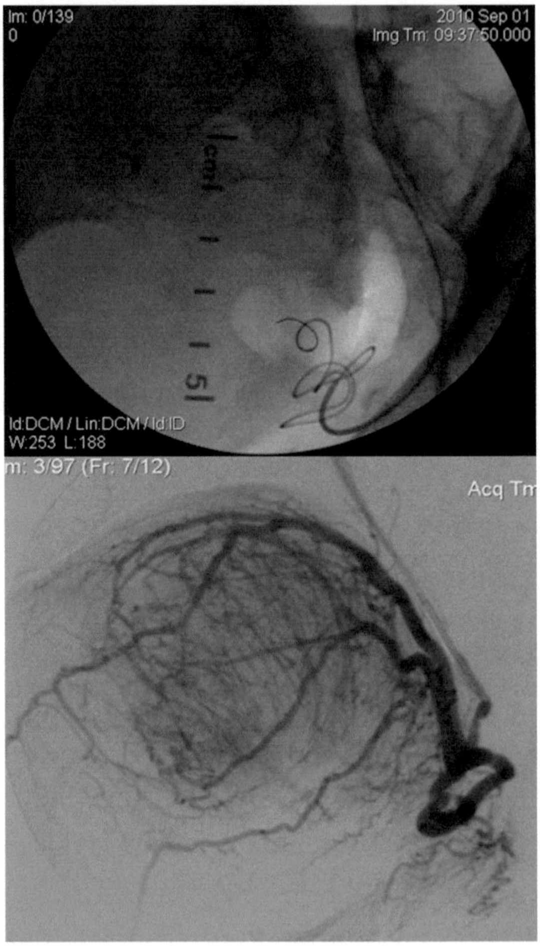

Figure 1.
Uterus myoma straight vessels.

conducted under the Helsinki Declaration. After detailed information of the participants regarding treatment options by the gynecologist and the invasive radiologist, written consent from every single one of the participants was obtained. Study participants were admitted to the University Obstetrics and Gynecology Clinic one day before the uterine artery embolization and underwent laboratory tests. On the procedure day they were receiving intravenous chemoprophylaxis and in particular iv Augmentin 600 mg and iv Metronidazole 1 g, while four hours before the UAE a urinary catheter was placed. Following the procedure, all participants received additional analgesic treatment every 4 h (tramadol 100 mg) and were monitored at the Department of University Obstetrics and Gynecology.

The clinical results of the study were based on evaluations concerning the overall satisfaction of the patients, the relief of clinical symptoms, the need for reoperation and hysterectomy and the amenorrhea rates during the follow-up period, which varied from 1 to 12 months.

3.1 Exclusion criteria

Included were postmenopausal women, patients with severe co-morbidities, patients who wished to maintain their fertility, patients with a known allergy to the contrast agent used during the procedure, and patients with suspected malignancy.

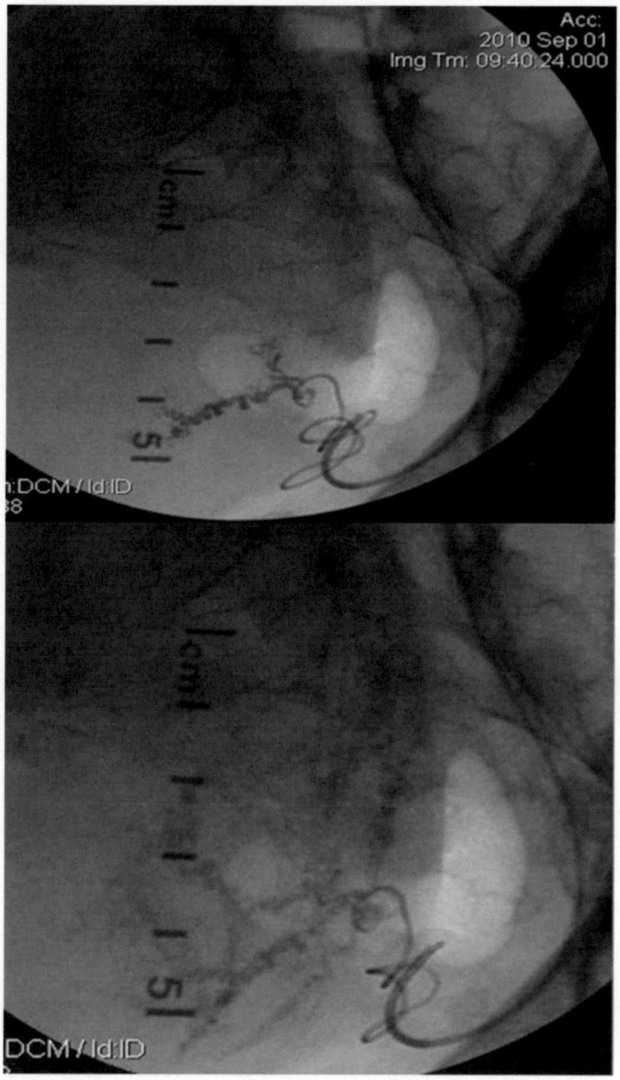

Figure 2.
Adenomyosis uteri spiral vessels.

There was no planned pregnancy or pelvic inflammation in the participants, while patients with only symptoms of back pain, asymptomatic, fibroid pendulum and rapidly improved size were excluded from the present study.

3.2 Study participants

A total of 64 patients met the inclusion criteria, with a mean admission age of 51 years (36–53). 40 patients (62.5%) were diagnosed with pure adenomyosis, 10 patients (15.62%) with focal adenomyosis (adenomyoma) and 14 patients (21.87%) with adenomyosis and fibroids. 50 participants (78%) had a history of pregnancy and childbirth in the past.

Reported symptoms included: dysmenorrhea (98%) with a mean VAS score of 8.8 (range 6–10), menorrhagia with menstrual clots (88%), menorrhagia without menstrual clots (53%) and urinary problems (12%). In terms of quality of life data, 76.5% of women complained of limited daily activities and low energy due to heavy menstrual bleeding, while 73.5% had problems with their sex life.

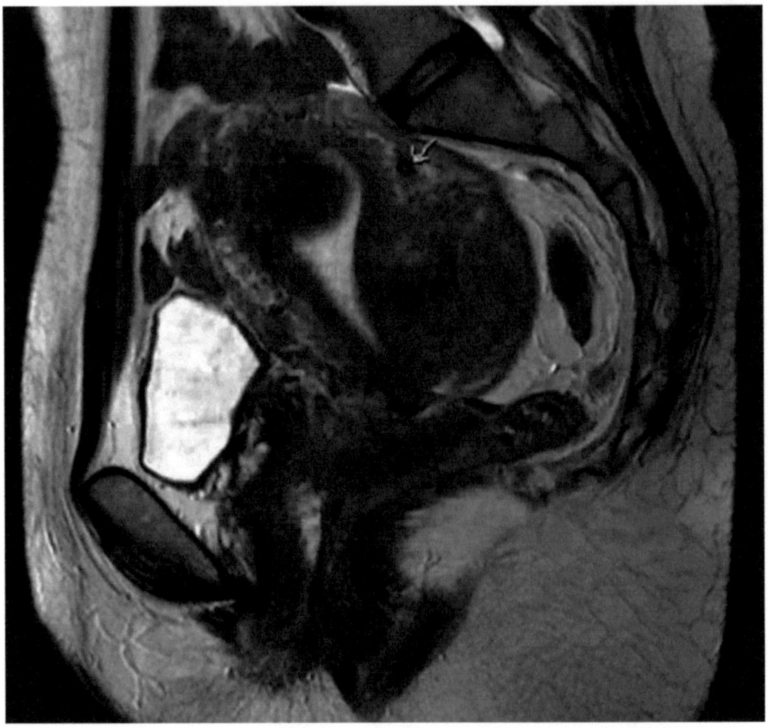

Figure 3.
Mixed type adenomyosis, myomas predominate, pressing and repelling the endometrium. MRI section, T2-WI, Sagital. Notice the increase in the width of the myometrial transition zone and hemosiderin granule (arrow) in the enlarged transition zone.

3.3 Results

According to our results, we confirm the following data:

Successful embolization (100%) was observed in all participants. On average, patients spent two days in the hospital, one day before the procedure and one on the day of the intervention. Elimination of clinical symptoms and reduction in pelvic pain intensity, assessed using VAS, was observed in 62 participants (96.87%). Pain in these cases decreased by an average of 7.5 points (from 8.2 to 1.0 points) during the follow-up period (from 1 to 12 months, average 3 months). Severe pain immediately after embolization and for approximately 24 h was observed in 8 cases with diffuse adenomyosis, 4 cases with adenomyoma and 2 cases with coexisting adenomyosis, in which analgesics and non-steroidal anti-inflammatory drugs were administered. In the majority of participants in our study, there were no significant complications associated with the procedure. However, in 4 participants (6.2%) recurrence of pain was observed within one to 2 months after embolism. In these cases, fractional dissolution is required, because submucosal fibroids coexist and adenomyosis diffuses. A postpartum neonatal ward of focal adenomyosis, sepsis, and surgical resection of necrotic sections was established, subject to the uterus. In no case was either reoperation or hysterectomy required. Restoration of normal menstruation was immediately observed in the subgroup of participants under 45 years of age. The other subgroup, which included participants over the age of 45, had normal menstruation. Only in 93% of cases immediately and only in 4 participants reported experience of the absence of menstruation for at least 3 months after embolization, resulting in the appearance of the period later after three months than in the other participants. In participants of the older participants over 45 years

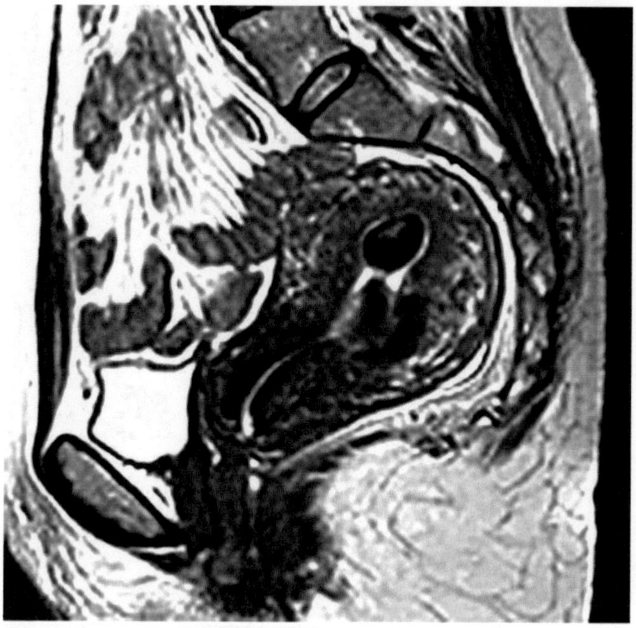

Figure 4.
MRI section, T2-WI, Sagital of the patient, six months after bilateral embolization. The myomas have completely degenerated and shrunk, however they continue to repel the endometrium to a lesser degree. The myometrial band anatomy has been restored to normal. The examination was performed with sections T2-WI, D-WI and T1-WI, simple and with spectral suppression of the magnetic fat signal, before and after intravenous administration of paramagnetic substance—situation after UAE 6 months ago. Degeneration, complete elimination of vasculitis and very significant further shrinkage of the two submucosal myomas, degeneration, ischemia and mild further shrinkage of the subarachnoid myoma of the anterior myometrium are observed, while the muscles of the fibroids are completely indistinguishable. The (normal) endometrium is slightly repelled by the two submucosal myomas. In the present examination, the uterus, which has been reduced in size, is presented with normal belt anatomy. Normal imaging of the cervix—a little free peritoneal liquid is shown in the Douglas pouch—the ovaries are normal—no pathological lymph nodes are not detected.

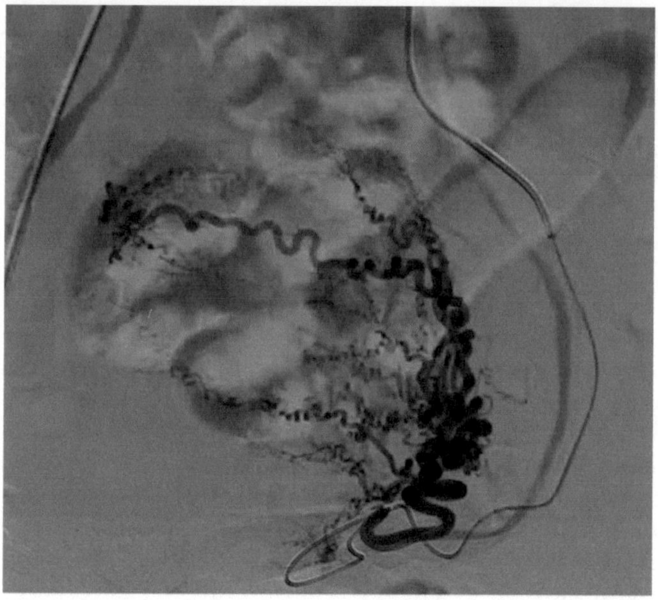

Figure 5.
Hyperelective catheterization and imaging before embolization of the left uterine artery, using a microcatheter. Observe the spiral vessels of adenomyosis and the straight lines of the myomas.

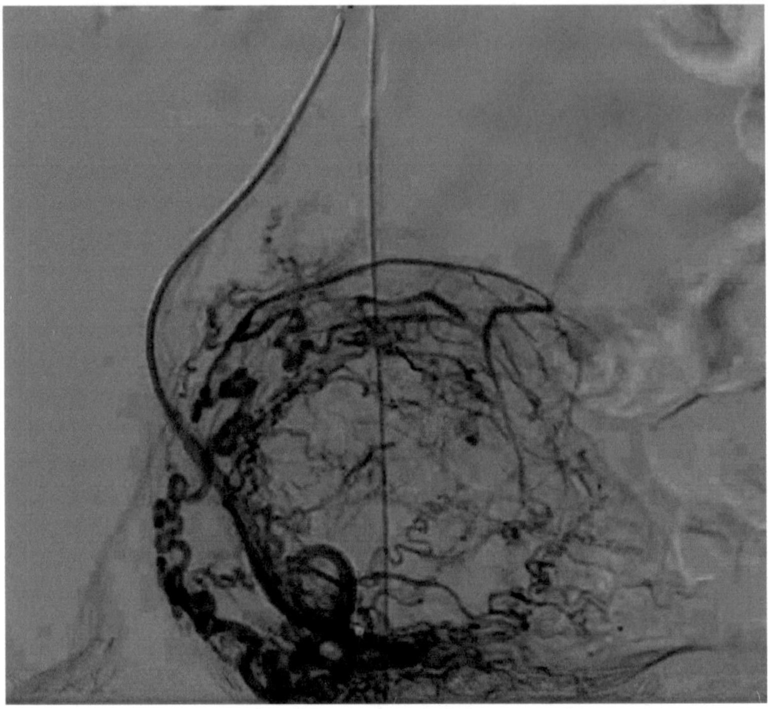

Figure 6.
Hyperelective catheterization and imaging before embolization of the right uterine artery, using a micro-catheter.

with a delayed onset of menstruation, low levels of AMH were established depending on biological age. Based on the findings of the MRI, partial or complete restoration of the normal zone anatomy in the uterus was confirmed after 6 months. All participants reported a decrease in menstrual bleeding and consequently improvement of everyday life quality. In one woman aged 49 years old, the decrease was not satisfactory and she underwent two months of analgesics therapy and after that the clinical symptoms were successfully improved. In our participants, the avoidance of hysterectomy was achieved in 100% of the women. All participants reported to be very or fairly satisfied with the results and would recommend this treatment to colleagues and friends.

4. Discussion

Adenomyosis is reasonable, although it has not been proven, that matrices with adenomyosis are deficient in activated T-cells, with the result that the basal endometrium in adenomyosis has an advantage in terms of growth potential over non-adenomyotic and lymphoid-rich basal formations. The adenomyosis led to reducing the junctional zone thickness whereas the latter results in the reduction of uterine volume. It remains a major problem that the diagnosis is based on its variable presentation and common coexistence of other gynecologic disorders like fibroids or endometriosis. Growth of adenomyosis focus proved due to contrast-enhanced MRI and TVUS are recommended currently as the most accurate imaging techniques for the diagnosis of the disease. The classical surgical procedure, hysterectomy, is recommended as the only definite treatment modus, while the other treatment alternatives medical and UAE are widely implemented and exist controversially reports [94–98].

Both treatments are reported to be successful, especially in the short term, but there are some long-term reports of UAE adenomyosis treatment being poor in success rate and reaching almost 50% of patients receiving treatment without reporting clinical improvement. Regarding the previously published reports, a recurrence rate of 38% was reported, satisfactory life results were observed in 76% of the participants. However, the question remains unanswered whether such an abnormality is necessarily associated with acquired "morbidity" of the myometrium or whether it is an independent condition for the development of adenomyosis. The exact cause of hyperplasia-hypertrophy of the myometrium, located around the deep foci of the endometrium, is not known [94–98].

Myometrial hyperplasia-hypertrophy may indicate either an attempt to control endometrial penetration or simply represent bundles of smooth muscle fibers displaced by the expanding endometrium. After examination, by immunohistochemical technique, it was found that the myometrium, which surrounds the ectopic endometrium either diffuse (adenomyosis) or focal (adenomyoma), does not show abnormalities. Smooth muscle cells in adenomyotic foci, normal myometrium and leiomyomas, whether or not coexisting with adenomyosis, are rich in actin and desmin [94–98]. Several experimental "models" have been reported to study the pathogenesis of adenomyosis. In one of them, endometrial grafts of the anterior pituitary gland in mice led to the development of adenomyosis [98–100]. Prolactin may amplify this, as the uterine horn that did not contain isografts showed relatively less development of adenomyosis. In this experimental model ovarian resection was prevented, while benzoic estradiol favored the development of adenomyosis.

In another mouse model, which received high doses of diethylstilbestrol (DES) during fetal life, adenomyosis developed. These genera of mice appear to be prone to developing adenomyosis when there are high concentrations of prolactin, estrogen and progestogens. More recently, other researchers have induced adenomyosis in uncastrated rats with hyperprolactinaemia [98–104].

The researchers argued that high concentrations of prolactin cause degeneration of the myometrium, with the concomitant presence of ovarian steroids, which leads to its weakening, resulting in the invasion of the basal layer of the endometrium. Also of great interest were the observations of Mori and Nagasawa in mice, in which the penetration of stromal fibroblasts along the branches of the myometrial blood vessels preceded the invasion of the endometrial glands [105].

In another study, Sakamoto et al., caused severe adenomyosis of the uterus in mice by placing ectopic anterior pituitary lobe isografts [106]. DNA synthesis-related activities and related enzymes, such as thymidyl synthetase and thymidine kinase, were significantly increased in adenomyosis matrices, compared with controls in the control group. In the same experimental model, it was found that finding low molecular weight metalloproteinases plays a role in the development of adenomyosis, at the level of gene transcription, activation and repression [99–108]. Specific experimental observations suggest that hereditary factors may be involved in the pathogenesis of adenomyosis. For example, the matrices of recombinant SMXA mice automatically develop adenomyosis-like histological changes and contain tenascin around the adenomyotic glands [100–108]. These observations, together with the biological properties of tenascin, reinforce the view of the endometrial origin of adenomyosis and the idea of endometrial penetration into the myometrium, which is genetically predisposed.

Also, compared to SMXA mice, the matrices of F1 mice, a genus found between SMXA and NJL, contain even more obvious spontaneous changes, resembling human adenomyosis. It should be noted, however, that it has not yet been determined whether heredity is an important factor in the development of adenomyosis in humans [100–108]. The early development of adenomyosis from remnants of Müller's ducts, in positions outside the uterus, is enhanced by the finding of adenomyosis in the rectal septum [100–108]. In this anatomical position can be found endometrial glands and layers, which are associated with hypertrophy of the adjacent smooth muscle fibers and form adenomyotic nodules [100–108]. Although, these nodules can develop as a result of penetration of the peritoneal endometriosis of their origin from remnants of Müller's resources. Thus, according to Nisolle and Donnez, in most cases, adenomyotic nodules are located deep in the septum and in some cases in the muscular layer of the rectum, away from the pelvic peritoneum [106–108]. The co-expression of vimentin and cytokeratin in the endometrium, when it is located in the endometrial cavity and when it is located in adenomyotic foci, is a typical feature of tissue, derived from Müller's ducts. Morphologically and in terms of receptor content, adenomyosis of the atrial septum is similar to that of the myometrium, including poor or no response to the post-ovulatory effect of progesterone. Despite the high doses of progestogens in women with rectal adenomyosis to induce secretory differentiation, hormone therapy has poor results. The definitive treatment of the rectal lesions with surgery also suggests the existence of a metaplastic process from the beginning, from remnants of Müller's ducts in this position, despite the implantation and penetration by peritoneal endometriosis [109–119].

Therefore, as the pathogenetic mechanisms of adenomyosis remain unclear, more studies are needed to reveal the pathophysiology of the disease. In the present study, all patients presented improvement in menorrhagia and had less blood loss during menstruation, while the effectiveness of the method appeared to be higher than that of other conservative surgeries such as intra-myometrial resection/excision and adenoectomy and laparoscopic myometrial electrocoagulation [119–125]. Radical surgery such as hysterectomy was eventually avoided in all participants, in 100% of the 64 patients. We did not observe the occurrence of permanent menopause, except in 0.6% of the participants, while transient amenorrhea within the first 3 months, occurred in the subgroup over the age of 45 years [119–125]. Premature menopause induction and subclinical reduction of ovarian functional reserve after the UAE is a known complication of this procedure, however, we have not observed any cases [119–125]. We know that our study has limitations and that the small sample size precludes a more detailed statistical analysis. Also, when adenomyosis coexists with uterine fibroids, it is very difficult to determine if the symptoms are caused by adenomyosis or the other. The incidence of pure adenomyosis is relatively low and due to a rare condition, individuals with co-existing fibroids were included [119–125].

5. Conclusions

In conclusion, despite the small number of participants, our preliminary study showed promising results with a very high rate of satisfied patients confirming that UAE might be a safe and effective method of treatment for premenopausal women with symptomatic adenomyosis in different if occurs with or without fibroids. It is a non-amputating treatment, alternative to hysterectomy UAE, for the treatment of symptomatic adenomyosis, when conservative treatment fails associated with few complications and allowed an option for the new session for recurrent disease.

Conflict of interest

None.

Notes/thanks/other declarations

I would like to many thanks to Emeritus Professor George Iatrakis for his scientific helpful contribution.

Author details

Panagiotis Tsikouras[1*], Fotini Gaitatzi[1], Stefani Filiou[1], Spyridon Michalopoulos[1], Aggeliki Gerede[1], Tsalikidis Christos[3], Stefanos Zervoudis[2], Anastasia Bothou[1], Xanthi Vatsidou[1], Anna Chalkidou[1], Georgios Dragoutsos[1], Ioannis Tsirkas[1], Konstantinos Nikolettos[1], Alexios Alexiou[1], Irine Babageorgaka[1], Natalia Sachnova[1], Nikolaos Panagiotopoulos[1], Theopi Nalbanti[1], Panagiotis Simeonidis[1], Nektaria Kritsotaki[1], Chrysovalantis Stylianou[4], Anastasios Vasilopoulos[4], Sebaidin Perende[3], Panagiotis Peitsidis[1], Nikolaos Nikolettos[1] and Vasileios Souftas[4]

1 Department of Obstetrics and Gynecology, Democritus University of Thrace, Alexandroupolis, Greece

2 Technological Educational Institute of Athens and Rea Maternity Hospital, Athens, Greece

3 Second Department of Surgery, University Hospital of Alexandroupolis, Democritus University of Thrace, Alexandroupolis, Greece

4 Department of Interventional Radiology, Democritus University of Thrace, Alexandroupolis, Greece

*Address all correspondence to: tsikouraspanagiotis@gmail.com

References

[1] Matalliotakis IM, Kourtis AI, Panidis DK. Adenomyosis. Obstetrics and Gynecology Clinics of North America. 2003;**30**(1):63-82, viii

[2] Siegler AM, Camilien L. Adenomyosis. The Journal of Reproductive Medicine. 1994;**39**(11):841-853

[3] Kissler S, Gaetje R, Siebzehnruebl E, Kaufmann M. New aspects in diagnosis and therapy of endometriosis. Zentralblatt für Gynäkologie. 2004; **126**(5):299-302 Review

[4] Ben Hamouda S, Ouerdiane N, Ben Zina H, et al. Adenomyosis at hysterectomy. La Tunisie Médicale. 2007;**85**(7):559-562

[5] Levgur MJ. Diagnosis of adenomyosis: A review. Reproductive Medicine. 2007;**52**(3):177-193

[6] Kissler S, Zangos S, Kohl J, et al. Duration of dysmenorrhoea and extent of adenomyosis visualised by magnetic resonance imaging. European Journal of Obstetrics, Gynecology, and Reproductive Biology. 2008;**137**(2): 204-209

[7] Adamyan L, Aznaurova Y, Stepanian A, et al. Gene expression signature of endometrial samples from women with and without endometriosis. Journal of Minimally Invasive Gynecology. 2021;**S1553-4650**(21): 00170-00179

[8] Bernardi M, Lazzeri L, Perelli F, et al. Dysmenorrhea and related disorders. F1000Research. 2017;**6**:1645. DOI: 10.12688/f1000research.11682.1. eCollection 2017

[9] Yang TWS, Ahn JMLJY. The molecular basis of adenomyosis development. Journal of Embryo Transfer. 2018;**33**(1):49-54. DOI: 10.12750/JET.2018.33.1.49

[10] Kay N, Huang C-Y, Shiu L-Y, et al. Neutralization improves pregnancy outcomes by restoring endometrial receptivity in mice with adenomyosis. Reproductive Sciences. 2021;**28**(3): 877-887

[11] Benagiano G, Brosens I. History of adenomyosis. Best Practice & Research: Clinical Obstetrics & Gynaecology. 2006;**20**(4):449-463

[12] Benagiano G, Brosens I, Lippi D. The history of endometriosis. Gynecologic and Obstetric Investigation. 2014; **78**(1):1-9

[13] Tamai K, Koyama T, Umeoka S, et al. Spectrum of MR features in adenomyosis. Best Practice & Research. Clinical Obstetrics & Gynaecology. 2006;**20**(4):583-602

[14] Marcus CC. Relationship of adenomyosis uteri to endometrial hyperplasia and endometrial carcinoma. American Journal of Obstetrics and Gynecology. 1961;**82**:408-416

[15] Bird CC, McElin TW, Manalo-Estrella P. The elusive adenomyosis of the uterus—Revisited. American Journal of Obstetrics & Gynecology. 1972;**112**(5):583-593

[16] Hudelist G, Keckstein J, Wright JT. The migrating adenomyoma: Past views on the etiology of adenomyosis and endometriosis. Fertility and Sterility. 2009;**92**(5):1536-1543

[17] Benagiano G, Brosens I, Habiba M. Structural and molecular features of the endomyometrium in endometriosis and adenomyosis. Human Reproduction Update. 2014;**20**(3):386-402

[18] Owolabi TO, Strickler RC. Adenomyosis: A neglected diagnosis. Obstetrics and Gynecology. 1977;**50**(4): 424-427

[19] Upson K, Missmer SA. Epidemiology of adenomyosis. Seminars in Reproductive Medicine. 2020;**38**(2-03):89-107

[20] Yu O, Schulze-Rath R, Grafton J, et al. Adenomyosis incidence, prevalence and treatment: United States population-based study 2006-2015. American Journal of Obstetrics and Gynecology. 2020;**223**(1):94

[21] Vercellini P, Viganò P, Somigliana E, et al. Adenomyosis: Epidemiological factors. Best Practice & Research. Clinical Obstetrics & Gynaecology. 2006;**20**(4):465-477. Review

[22] Upson K, Missmer SA. Epidemiology of adenomyosis. Seminars in Reproductive Medicine. 2020; **38**(2-03):89-107

[23] Naphatthalung W, Cheewadhanaraks S. Prevalence of endometriosis among patients with adenomyosis and/or myoma uteri scheduled for a hysterectomy. Journal of the Medical Association of Thailand. 2012;**95**(9):1136-1140

[24] Upson K, Missmer SA. Epidemiology of adenomyosis. Seminars in Reproductive Medicine. 2020;**38**(2-03):89-107

[25] Milingos S, Protopapas A, Drakakis P, et al. Laparoscopic management of patients with endometriosis and chronic pelvic pain. Annals of the New York Academy of Sciences. 2003;**997**:269-273

[26] Vercellini P, Trespidi L, De Giorgi O, et al. Endometriosis and pelvic pain: Relation to disease stage and localization. Fertility and Sterility. 1996;**65**(2):299-304

[27] Ridley JH. The validity of Sampson's theory of endometriosis. American Journal of Obstetrics and Gynecology. 1961;**82**:777-782

[28] Vollmer G, Siegal GP, Chiquet-Ehrismann R, Lightner VA, Arnholdt H, Knuppen R. Tenascin expression in the human endometrium and in endometrial adenocarcinomas. Laboratory Investigation. 1990;**62**(6): 725-730

[29] Matsuda M, Sasabe H, Adachi Y, et al. Increased invasion activity of endometrial stromal cells and elevated expression of matrix metalloproteinase messenger RNA in the uterine tissues of mice with experimentally induced adenomyosis. American Journal of Obstetrics and Gynecology. 2001;**185**(6):1374-1380

[30] Goumenou AG, Arvanitis DA, Spandidos DA. Loss of heterozygosity in adenomyosis on hMSH2, hMLH1, p16Ink4 and GALT loci. International Journal of Molecular Medicine. 2000; **6**(6):667-671

[31] Bulun SE, Yildiz S, Adli M, et al. Adenomyosis pathogenesis: Insights from next-generation sequencing. Human Reproduction. 2021;**27**(6):1086-1097. DOI: 10.1093/humupd/dmab017

[32] Lacheta J. Uterine adenomyosis: Pathogenesis, diagnostics, symptomatology and treatment. Ceská Gynekologie. 2019;**84**(3):240-246. Review

[33] Vannuccini S, Tosti C, Carmona F, et al. Pathogenesis of adenomyosis: An update on molecular mechanisms. Reproductive Biomedicine Online. 2017;**35**(5):592-601

[34] Antero MF, Ayhan A, Segars J, Shih IM. Pathology and pathogenesis of adenomyosis. Seminars in Reproductive Medicine. 2020;**38**(2-03):108-118

[35] Guo SW. The pathogenesis of adenomyosis vis-a-vis endometriosis. Journal of Clinical Medicine. 2020; **9**(2):485

[36] Antero MF, Ayhan A, Segars J, Shih IM. Pathology and pathogenesis of adenomyosis. Seminars in Reproductive Medicine. 2020;**38**(2-03):108-118

[37] Zhai J, Vannuccini S, Petraglia F. et al, Adenomyosis: Mechanisms and pathogenesis. Seminars in Reproductive Medicine. 2020;**38**(2-03):129-143

[38] García-Solares J, Donnez J, Donnez O, et al. Pathogenesis of uterine adenomyosis: Invagination or metaplasia? Fertility and Sterility. 2018;**109**(3):371-379

[39] Langlois PL. The size of the normal uterus. The Journal of Reproductive Medicine. 1970;**4**(6):220-228

[40] Mark AS, Hricak H, Heinrichs LW, et al. Adenomyosis and leiomyoma: Differential diagnosis with MR imaging. Radiology. 1987;**163**(2):527-529

[41] Sandberg EC, Cohn F. Adenomyosis in the gravid uterus at term. American Journal of Obstetrics & Gynecology. 1962;**84**:1457-1465

[42] Azziz R. Adenomyosis in pregnancy. A review. Journal of Reproductive Medicine. 1986;**31**(4):224-227

[43] Parazzini F, Mais V, Cipriani S, et al. Determinants of adenomyosis in women who underwent hysterectomy for benign gynecological conditions: Results from a prospective multicentric study in Italy. European Journal of Obstetrics, Gynecology, and Reproductive Biology. 2009;**143**(2):103-106

[44] Song Y, Fazleabas AT. Endometrial organoids: A rising star for research on endometrial development and associated diseases. Reproductive Sciences. 2021;**28**(6):1626-1636. Review

[45] Zhu J, Mayr D, Kuhn C, Mahner S, et al. Prostaglandin E2 receptor EP1 in healthy and diseased human endometrium. Histochemistry and Cell Biology. 2018;**149**(2):153-160

[46] Ben Hamouda S, Ouerdiane N, Ben Zina H. et al, Adenomyosis at hysterectomy. La Tunisie Médicale. 2007;**85**(7):559-562

[47] Bergeron C, Amant F, Ferenczy A. Pathology and physiopathology of adenomyosis. Best Practice & Research. Clinical Obstetrics & Gynaecology. 2006;**20**(4):511-521. Review

[48] McLucas B. Diagnosis, imaging and anatomical classification of uterine fibroids. Best Practice & Research. Clinical Obstetrics & Gynaecology. 2008;**22**(4):627-642. Review

[49] Kishi Y, Shimada K, Fujii T, et al. Phenotypic characterization of adenomyosis occurring at the inner and outer myometrium. PLoS One. 2017;**12**(12):e0189522

[50] Azziz R. Adenomyosis: Current perspectives. Obstetrics and Gynecology Clinics of North America. 1989;**16**(1): 221-235. Review

[51] Graham KJ, Hulst FA, Vogelnest L, et al. Uterine adenomyosis in an orang-utan (Pongo abelii/pygmaeus). Australian Veterinary Journal. 2009;**87**(1):66-69. Review

[52] Basak S, Saha A. Adenomyosis: Still largely under-diagnosed. The Obstetrician and Gynaecologist. 2009;**29**(6):533-535

[53] Chapron C, Vannuccini S, Pistofidis G, Petraglia F. Diagnosing adenomyosis: An integrated clinical and imaging approach. Human Reproduction Update. 2020;**26**(3): 392-411

[54] Struble J, Reid S, Bedaiwy MA. Adenomyosis: A clinical review of a challenging gynecologic condition. Journal of Minimally Invasive Gynecology. 2016;**23**(2):164-185

[55] Munro MG. Classification and reporting systems for adenomyosis. Journal of Minimally Invasive Gynecology. 2020;**27**(2):296-308

[56] Vannuccini S, Petraglia F. Recent advances in understanding and

managing adenomyosis. F1000Research. 2019;**8**:F1000. Faculty Rev-283

[57] Panganamamula UR, Harmanli OH, Isik-Akbay EF, et al. Is prior uterine surgery a risk factor for adenomyosis? Obstetrics and Gynecology. 2004;**104**(5 Pt 1):1034-1038

[58] Kdous M, Ferchiou M, Zhioua F. Uterine adenomyosis, clinical and therapeutic study: About 87 cases. The Pan African Medical Journal. 2015;**22**:73

[59] Kilkku P, Erkkola R, Grönroos M. Non-specificity of symptoms related to adenomyosis. A prospective comparative survey. Acta Obstetricia et Gynecologica Scandinavica. 1984;**63**(3):229-231

[60] Peric H, Fraser IS. The symptomatology of adenomyosis. Best Practice & Research: Clinical Obstetrics & Gynaecology. 2006;**20**(4):547-555. DOI: 10.1016/j.bpobgyn.2006.01.006. Epub 2006 Mar 2

[61] Levgur M, Abadi MA, Tucker A. Adenomyosis: Symptoms, histology, and pregnancy terminations. Obstetrics and Gynecology. 2000;**95**(5):688-691

[62] Morita M, Asakawa Y, Kubo H, et al. Laparoscopic excision of myometrial adenomyomas in patients with adenomyosis uteri and main symptoms of severe dysmenorrhea and hypermenorrhea. The Journal of the American Association of Gynecologic Laparoscopists. 2004;**11**(1):86-89

[63] Parrott E, Butterworth M, Greaves P, et al. Adenomyosis—A result of disordered stromal differentiation. American Journal of Pathology. 2001; **159**(2):623-630

[64] Nisolle M, Donnez J. Peritoneal endometriosis, ovarian endometriosis, and adenomyotic nodules of the rectovaginal septum are three different entities. Fertility and Sterility. 1997;**68**(4): 585-596

[65] Wilde S, Scott-Barrett S. Radiological appearances of uterine fibroids. Indian Journal of Radiology and Imaging. 2009;**19**(3):222-231

[66] Takeuchi M, Matsuzaki K. Adenomyosis: Usual and unusual imaging manifestations, pitfalls, and problem-solving MR imaging techniques. Radiographics. 2011;**31**(1): 99-115. Review

[67] Marshak RH. Eliasoph The roentgen findings in adenomyosis. Journal of Radiology. 1955;**64**(6):846-851

[68] Siedler D, Laing FC, Wing VW, et al. Uterine adenomyosis. A difficult sonographic diagnosis. Journal of Ultrasound in Medicine. 1987;**6**(7): 345-349

[69] Mark AS, Hricak H, Heinrichs LW, Hendrickson MR, Winkler ML, Bachica JA, et al. Adenomyosis and leiomyoma: Differential diagnosis with MR imaging. Radiology. 1987;**163**(2): 527-529

[70] Takahashi K, Kijima S, Yoshino K, et al. Differential diagnosis between leiomyomata uteri and adenomyosis using CA 125 as a new tumor marker of ovarian carcinoma. Nihon Sanka Fujinka Gakkai Zasshi. 1985;**37**(4): 591-595

[71] Babacan A, Kizilaslan C, Gun I, Muhcu M, Mungen E, Atay V. CA 125 and other tumor markers in uterine leiomyomas and their association with lesion characteristics. International Journal of Clinical and Experimental Medicine. 2014;**7**(4):1078-1083

[72] Halila H, Suikkari AM, Seppälä M. The effect of hysterectomy on serum CA 125 levels in patients with adenomyosis and uterine fibroids. Human Reproduction. 1987;**2**(3):265-266

[73] Zhou Y, Wu B, Li H. The value of serum CA125 assays in the diagnosis of

uterine adenomyosis. Zhonghua Fu Chan Ke Za Zhi. 1996;**31**(10):590-593

[74] Masahashi T, Matsuzawa K, Ohsawa M, Narita O, Asai T, Ishihara M. Serum CA 125 levels in patients with endometriosis: Changes in CA 125 levels during menstruation. Obstetrics and Gynecology. 1988;**72**(3 Pt 1):328-331

[75] Bergeron C, Amant F, Ferenczy A. Pathology and physiopathology of adenomyosis. Best Practice & Research. Clinical Obstetrics & Gynaecology. 2006;**20**(4):511-521. Epub 2006 Mar 24 Review

[76] Babacan A, Kizilaslan C, Gun I, Muhcu M, Mungen E, Atay V. CA 125 and other tumor markers in uterine leiomyomas and their association with lesion characteristics. International Journal of Clinical and Experimental Medicine. 2014;**7**(4):1078-1083

[77] Levy G, Hill MJ, Plowden TC, Catherino WH, Armstrong AY. Biomarkers in uterine leiomyoma. Fertility and Sterility. 2013;**99**(4): 1146-1152

[78] Ayas S, Bayraktar M, Gürbüz A, et al. Uterine junctional zone thickness, cervical length and bioelectrical impedance analysis of body composition in women with endometriosis. Balkan Medical Journal. 2012;**29**(4):410-413

[79] Yang CC, Tseng JY, Wang PH. Uterus didelphys with cervical agenesis associated with adenomyosis, a leiomyoma and ovarian endometriosis. A case report. Journal o Reproductive Medicine. 2002;**47**(11):936-938

[80] Woodruff JD, Erozan YS, Genadry R. Adenocarcinoma arising in adenomyosis detected by atypical cytology. Obstetrics and Gynecology. 1986;**67**(1):145-148

[81] Kay S, Frable WJ, Goplerud DR. Endometrial carcinoma arising in a large polypoid adenomyoma of the uterus. International Journal of Gynecological Pathology. 1988;**7**(4):391-398

[82] Yen CF, Huang SJ, Liao SK, et al. Molecular characteristics of the endometrium in uterine adenomyosis and its biochemical microenvironment. Reproductive Sciences. 2017;**24**(10): 1346-1361

[83] Özkan ZS, Kumbak B, Cilgin H, Simsek M, Turk BA. Coexistence of adenomyosis in women operated for benign gynecological diseases. Gynecological Endocrinology. 2012;**28**(3): 212-215

[84] Donnez J, Nisolle M, Casanas-Roux F, Bassil S, Anaf V. Rectovaginal septum, endometriosis or adenomyosis: Laparoscopic management in a series of 231 patients. Human Reproduction. 1995;**10**(3): 630-635

[85] Leyendecker G, Kunz G, Kissler S, Wildt L. Adenomyosis and reproduction. Best Practice & Research: Clinical Obstetrics & Gynaecology. 2006;**20**(4):523-546

[86] Chen M, Luo L, Wang Q, et al. Impact of gonadotropin-releasing hormone agonist pre-treatment on the cumulative live birth rate in infertile women with adenomyosis treated with IVF/ICSI: A retrospective Cohort study. Frontiers in Endocrinology (Lausanne). 2020;**11**:318

[87] Leyendecker G, Kunz G, Wildt L. Adenomyosis and reproduction. Best Practice & Research: Clinical Obstetrics & Gynaecology. 2006;**20**(4): 523-546

[88] Katsikogiannis N, Tsaroucha A, Simopoulos C. Rectal endometriosis causing colonic obstruction and concurrent endometriosis of the appendix: A case report. Journal of Medical Case Reports. 2011;**5**:320

[89] Li JJ, Chung JPW, Duan H. The investigation and management of adenomyosis in women who wish to improve or preserve fertility. BioMed Research International. 2018;**2018**: 6832685

[90] Tamura H, Kishi H, Kitade M, et al. Clinical outcomes of infertility treatment for women with adenomyosis in Japan. Reproductive Medicine and Biology. 2017;**16**(3):276-282

[91] Di Spiezio SA, Calagna G, Santangelo F, et al. The role of hysteroscopy in the diagnosis and treatment of adenomyosis. BioMed Research International. 2017;**2017**: 2518396

[92] Leyendecker G, Bilgicyildirim A, Inacker M, et al. Adenomyosis and endometriosis. Re-visiting their association and further insights into the mechanisms of auto-traumatisation. An MRI study. Archives of Gynecology and Obstetrics. 2015;**291**(4):917-932

[93] Ferrari F, Arrigoni F, Miccoli A, et al. Effectiveness of Magnetic Resonance-guided Focused Ultrasound Surgery (MRgFUS) in the uterine adenomyosis treatment: Technical approach and MRI evaluation. La Radiologia Medica. 2016;**121**(2):153-161

[94] Gao Y, Shan S, Zhao X, et al. Clinical efficacy of adenomyomectomy using "H" type incision combined with Mirena in the treatment of adenomyosis. Medicine (Baltimore). 2019;**98**(11): e14579

[95] Kishi Y, Yabuta M. The benefit of adenomyomectomy on fertility outcomes in women with rectovaginal endometriosis with coexisting adenomyosis. Gynecology and Minimally Invasive Therapy. 2017;**6**(1):20-24

[96] de Bruijn AM, Smink M, Hehenkamp WJK, et al. Uterine artery embolization for symptomatic adenomyosis: 7-year clinical follow-up using UFS-Qol questionnaire. Cardiovascular and Interventional Radiology. 2017;**40**(9):1344-1350

[97] de Bruijn AM, Smink M, Lohle PNM, et al. Uterine artery embolization for the treatment of adenomyosis: A systematic review and meta-analysis. Journal of Vascular and Interventional Radiology. 2017;**28**(12): 1629-1642.e1

[98] Dessouky R, Gamil SA, Nada MG, Mousa R, Libda Y. Management of uterine adenomyosis: Current trends and uterine artery embolization as a potential alternative to hysterectomy. Insights Imaging. 2019 Apr 27;**10**(1):48. DOI: 10.1186/s13244-019-0732-8

[99] Alvi FA, Glaser LM, Chaudhari A, et al. New paradigms in the conservative surgical and interventional management of adenomyosis. Current Opinion in Obstetrics & Gynecology. 2017;**29**(4): 240-248

[100] Lefebvre G, Vilos G, Allaire C, et al. The management of uterine leiomyomas. Clinical Practice Gynaecology Committee, Society for Obstetricians and Gynaecologists of Canada. Journal of Obstetrics and Gynaecology Canada. 2003;**25**(5): 396-418; quiz 419-22

[101] Dueholm M. Minimally invasive treatment of adenomyosis. Best Practice & Research. Clinical Obstetrics & Gynaecology. 2018;**51**:119-137

[102] Smeets AJ, Nijenhuis RJ, Boekkooi PF, et al. Long-term follow-up of uterine artery embolization for symptomatic adenomyosis. Cardiovascular and Interventional Radiology. 2012;**35**(4):815-819

[103] Liang E, Brown B, Rachinsky M. A clinical audit on the efficacy and safety of uterine artery embolisation for

symptomatic adenomyosis: Results in 117 women. The Australian & New Zealand Journal of Obstetrics & Gynaecology. 2018;**58**(4):454-459

[104] Marshburn PB, Matthews ML, Hurst BS. Uterine artery embolization as a treatment option for uterine myomas. Obstetrics and Gynecology Clinics of North America. 2006;**33**(1):125-144 Review

[105] Mori T, Nagasawa H. Mechanisms of development of prolactin-induced adenomyosis in mice. Acta Anatomica (Basel). 1983;**116**(1):46-54

[106] Sakamoto A. Subserosal adenomyosis: A possible variant of pelvic endometriosis. American Journal of Obstetrics and Gynecology. 1991;**165**(1):198-201

[107] Donnez J, Nisolle M, Smoes P, et al. Peritoneal endometriosis and "endometriotic" nodules of the rectovaginal septum are two different entities. Fertility and Sterility. 1996;**66**(3):362-368

[108] Nisolle M, Donnez J. Peritoneal endometriosis, ovarian endometriosis, and adenomyotic nodules of the rectovaginal septum are three different entities. Fertility and Sterility. 1997;**68**(4):585-596

[109] de Bruijn AM, Smink M, Lohle PNM, et al. Uterine artery embolization for the treatment of adenomyosis: A systematic review and meta-analysis. Journal of Vascular and Interventional Radiology. 2017;**28**(12):1629-1642.e1. Review

[110] Sharara FI, Kheil MH, Feki A, et al. Current and prospective treatment of adenomyosis. Journal of Clinical Medicine. 2021;**10**(15):3410

[111] Mikos T, Lioupis M, Grimbizis GF, et al. The outcome of fertility-sparing and nonfertility-sparing surgery for the treatment of adenomyosis. A systematic review and meta-analysis. Journal of Minimally Invasive Gynecology. 2020;**27**(2):309-331.e3

[112] Soave I, Wenger JM, Pluchino N, et al. Treatment options and reproductive outcome for adenomyosis-associated infertility. Current Medical Research and Opinion. 2018;**34**(5):839-849

[113] Oliveira MAP, Crispi CP Jr, Brollo LC, et al. Surgery in adenomyosis. Archives of Gynecology and Obstetrics. 2018;**297**(3):581-589

[114] Rocha TP, Andres MP, Borrelli GM, Abrão MS. Fertility-sparing treatment of adenomyosis in patients with infertility: A systematic review of current options. Reproductive Sciences. 2018;**25**(4):480-486

[115] Marques ALS, Andres MP, Kho RM, et al. Is high-intensity focused ultrasound effective for the treatment of adenomyosis? A systematic review and meta-analysis. Journal of Minimally Invasive Gynecology. 2020;**27**(2):332-343

[116] Pyra K, Szmygin M, Szmygin H, Bèrczi V, Kidzinski R, Jargiello T, et al. Endovascular embolization as a treatment for symptomatic adenomyosis—Results of preliminary study. Ginekologia Polska. 2021. DOI: 10.5603/GP.a2021.0136

[117] Kim MD, Kim S, Kim NK, et al. Long-term results of uterine artery embolization for symptomatic adenomyosis. AJR. American Journal of Roentgenology. 2007;**188**(1):176-181

[118] de Bruijn AM, Ankum WM, Reekers, et al. Uterine artery embolization vs hysterectomy in the treatment of symptomatic uterine fibroids: 10-year outcomes from the randomized EMMY trial. American Journal of Obstetrics and Gynecology. 2016;**215**(6):745.e1-745.e12

[119] Gupta JK, Sinha A, Lumsden MA, et al. Uterine artery embolization for symptomatic uterine fibroids. Cochrane Database of Systematic Reviews. 2014;(12):CD005073. Review

[120] Yang W, Liu M, Liu L, et al. Uterine-sparing laparoscopic pelvic plexus ablation, uterine artery occlusion, and partial adenomyomectomy for adenomyosis. Journal of Minimally Invasive Gynecology. 2017;**24**(6): 940-945

[121] Kang L, Gong J, Cheng Z, et al. Clinical application and midterm results of laparoscopic partial resection of symptomatic adenomyosis combined with uterine artery occlusion. Journal of Minimally Invasive Gynecology. 2009;**16**(2):169-173

[122] Peters A, Rindos NB, Guido RS, et al. Uterine-sparing laparoscopic resection of accessory cavitated uterine masses. Journal of Minimally Invasive Gynecology. 2018;**25**(1):24-25

[123] Oliveira MAP, Crispi CP Jr, Brollo LC, et al. Surgery in adenomyosis. Archives of Gynecology and Obstetrics. 2018;**297**(3):581-589

[124] Kwack JY, Kwon YS. Kaohsiung conservative surgery of diffuse adenomyosis with TOUA: Single surgeon experience of one hundred sixteen cases and report of fertility outcomes. Journal of Medical Sciences. 2018;**34**(5):290-294

[125] Chen D, Ai G, Yang W, et al. Laparoscopic uterine artery occlusion combined with uterine-sparing pelvic plexus block and partial adenomyomectomy for adenomyosis: A video case report. Journal of Minimally Invasive Gynecology. 2021;**S1553-4650**(21):00237-00235

Chapter 7

Applying Machine Learning Algorithms to Predict Endometriosis Onset

Ewa J. Kleczyk, Tarachand Yadav and Stalin Amirtharaj

Abstract

Endometriosis is a commonly occurring progressive gynecological disorder, in which tissues similar to the lining of the uterus grow on other parts of the female body, including ovaries, fallopian tubes, and bowel. It is one of the primary causes of pelvic discomfort and fertility challenges in women. The actual cause of the endometriosis is still undetermined. As a result, the objective of the chapter is to identify the drivers of endometriosis' diagnoses via leveraging selected advanced machine learning (ML) algorithms. The primary risks of infertility and other health complications can be minimized to a greater extent if a likelihood of endometriosis could be predicted well in advance. Logistic regression (LR) and eXtreme Gradient Boosting (XGB) algorithms leveraged 36 months of medical history data to demonstrate the feasibility. Several direct and indirect features were identified as important to an accurate prediction of the condition onset, including selected diagnosis and procedure codes. Creating analytical tools based on the model results that could be integrated into the Electronic Health Records (EHR) systems and easily accessed by healthcare providers might aid the objective of improving the diagnostic processes and result in a timely and precise diagnosis, ultimately increasing patient care and quality of life.

Keywords: endometriosis, infertility, likelihood, logistic regression, machine learning, eXtreme gradient boosting, nomogram, odds ratio

1. Introduction

Recent advancements in artificial intelligence (AI) and machine learning (ML) have offered an opportunity for utilization of these advanced methodologies in the healthcare industry, while also at the same time improving upon the performance and accuracy benchmarks established by the classical statistical techniques [1]. A variety of ML techniques have been already applied to clinical data to examine a number of conditions and therapeutic areas, their onset, progression, and treatment options. In addition, deep learning algorithms such as convolutional neural network (CNN) have been employed in medical image data to predict disease onset and progression with even greater precision [2–5].

ML algorithms applied to a large amount of structured and unstructured data and combined with available data processing technology have already improved researchers' ability to mine the vast amount of data and assisted in making the patient healthcare decisions [6]. As a result of the high precision and robustness of

 IntechOpen

ML algorithms compared to the classical statistical methods, the insights derived from the application of these methods became important in driving the strategies and processes related to healthcare access, patient care, as well as disease diagnostics, healthcare trend forecasting, drug discovery, etc., thereby, further impacting the ability to reducing medical costs, shortening the time to diagnoses and treatment, and enhancing patients' quality of life and outcomes [7].

Endometriosis is one of the most commonly occurring disorders in women of menstruating age. Tissues, resembling the endometrium lining, grow on the outer part of the uterus and other organs of the pelvic area. The signs and symptoms differ across patients with some individuals experiencing mild symptoms, while others displaying moderate to severe signs. The most common symptoms of endometriosis include pain in the pelvic area, dysmenorrhea, and the inability to have children. Most commonly laparoscopy, surgery under general anesthesia, is performed to confirm the diagnosis of endometriosis [8]. Since it is an invasive procedure, it may not be suitable for all women. Laparoscopy is also quite expensive and women require a confirmation of a variety of indicatives of endometriosis before undergoing this procedure [9]. There are also a number of studies researching biomarkers of endometriosis via assessing endometrial tissue, uterine or menstrual fluids, immunological markers in blood or urine, gene expressions, etc. [10].

The availability of noninvasive methods to predict the likelihood of endometriosis could reduce the diagnostic delays and the number of women undergoing surgery unnecessarily, and thus avoiding unwanted complications and potential trauma [11]. In other research studies, researchers developed a new ensemble technique called GenomeForest that analyzed the gene expression data. The method systematically examined capabilities in classifying endometriosis and control samples, using both transcriptomics and methylomics data [12, 13].

Another research study developed symptom-based models that predicted the likelihood of endometriosis using logistic regression (LR). Symptomatic data including patient demographics, women's past medical history, obstetrics, family history, etc. were collected through a 25-item self-administered questionnaire [14]. Researchers also systematically applied selected ultrasound techniques in the diagnosis of endometriosis and concluded that these methods should remain the first-line procedures in the evaluation of patients with endometriosis [15].

In recent years, researchers aimed at developing CNN-based CAD systems that could classify endometrial lesions images obtained from hysteroscopy and evaluate the diagnostic performance of the model [16]. Their system slightly outperformed gynecologists in classifying endometrial lesion images. With a large number of diagnostic procedures, there is, however, no guaranteed treatment for endometriosis at this time. With an early diagnosis and available medical and surgical options; however, healthcare providers might be able to reduce the risks of potential complications and improve the quality of life for their patients [17, 18].

In the above research studies, researchers used either relatively small samples, or a limited number of variables to develop models or systems to predict the likelihood of endometriosis. The source of data represented mostly clinics and care providers in a controlled environment. There have been a limited amount of research studies performed thus far leveraging US-based patient-level claims data in predicting endometriosis. Claims data consist of the entire patient medical journey, such as diagnosis, procedures, prescriptions, physician, and patient demographics [19, 20]. In this chapter, US patient-level claims datasets at a transactional level were leveraged to develop accurate ML algorithms to predict the likelihood of endometriosis onset. Predicting the probability of endometriosis occurrence via leveraging the diagnosed patients' medical history might benefit both the diagnostics process as well as improved patients' quality of life. The LR and eXtreme Gradient Boosting

(XGB) algorithms were employed to identify the key drivers of endometriosis onset. An earlier version of this chapter is available on the Research Square website. The posting allowed for the dissemination of these important insights with the research community in advance, while at the same time, leveraging the received feedback to enhance the research design in this chapter.

2. Methodology overview

As mentioned earlier, the analysis design was described in the earlier version of the chapter available on the Research Square website. It leveraged the US healthcare claims patient-level database with the period from January 31, 2019 to December 31, 2019 [21]. Patients with a history of medical diagnosis ICD 10 codes for endometriosis were labeled as targets and the remaining patients were assigned as controls. As endometriosis is a women-only condition, female patients 18 and older were selected for the study target cohort. A control cohort, using a propensity matching algorithm, was built as a comparison group to the study targets. Thirty six (36) months of patients' medical history before the first condition event in 2019 were extracted for both cohorts. The US healthcare claims data included diagnosis, medical, procedural, surgical, and hospital codes, as well as medical treatments and therapies prescribed to patients. The dataset was presented at the transactional level to ensure proper capture of medical events longitudinally [21]. Several analytical approaches were employed for the analysis from the rules-based patient qualification criteria to ML algorithms to derive the probability of endometriosis onset. The healthcare claims patient-level dataset considered in the analysis represented healthcare claims sourced for the United States regions only.

2.1 Healthcare claims patient-level database

The US healthcare claims patient-level database is an anonymous longitudinal patient dataset often applied by healthcare organizations to derive insights [22, 23], while at the same time informing the effective treatment outcome options, patient access strategies, and areas for improvement in the diagnostic process [19]. The US healthcare claims patient-level database employed for this chapter consisted of medical, procedural, surgical, hospital, and prescriptions claims across all types of insurance payments and all geographic areas in the United States [24, 25]. The healthcare claims database overall covered more than 317 million active patients with over more than 17 years of medical health history and involved more than 1.9 million healthcare providers [25]. **Figure 1** presents the summary of information in the database.

2.2 Cohort selection

For this chapter, a sample of 314,101 confirmed endometriosis patients in 2019 in the US healthcare claims patient-level database was leveraged for the analysis. The patients were identified using predefined ICD 10 diagnosis codes (**Table 1**). Female patients of age 18 and older were identified for the target cohort. For the control cohort, a random sample of 3 million female patients with the same age specifications was selected from the database [21].

To define a control cohort of an equal size to the study target group, a 'propensity score matching' methodology was employed [18]. The algorithm selected the controls based on several similar characteristics or covariates. Covariates included patient age and medical history [26, 27]. **Table 2** presents the summary of the distribution comparison between the study target and control cohorts by age and

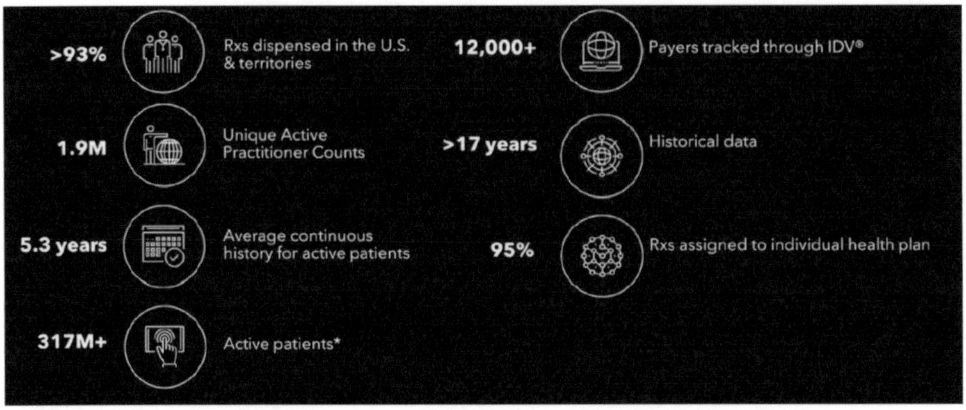

Figure 1.
Healthcare claims patient level database summary.

Diagnosis	Codes diagnosis long description
N80.0	Endometriosis of uterus
N80.1	Endometriosis of ovary
N80.2	Endometriosis of fallopian tube
N80.3	Endometriosis of pelvic peritoneum
N80.4	Endometriosis of rectovaginal septum and vagina
N80.5	Endometriosis of intestine
N80.6	Endometriosis in cutaneous scar
N80.8	Other endometriosis
N80.9	Endometriosis, unspecified

Table 1.
ICD 10 diagnosis codes of endometriosis.

Age group	Target (%)	Control (%)
18–24	6.45	6.55
25–34	25.01	25.24
35–44	37.57	37.08
45–54	23.13	23.18
55–64	6.22	6.31
65+	1.62	1.64
Region	**Target (%)**	**Control (%)**
South	39.90	39.90
Midwest	22.78	22.76
Northeast	18.82	18.84
West	17.02	17.02
Other	1.48	1.48

Table 2.
Comparison between target and control cohort by age and region respectively.

Census geographies. The patient age variable was created via grouping age ranges, while states were grouped into the US regions [21].

2.3 Data extraction

The next step in the analysis process was to pull the patients' medical history from the available information in the US healthcare claims patient-level database [21]. The event date for the target cohort was established for each individual in the study to ensure the extraction of the healthcare information before the first condition event. For the control cohort, the first activity in 2019 was leveraged as the event date [21].

The approach for the data extraction and the study target and control setup was the same as presented in the earlier version of the chapter available on Research Square. Using the medical event dates, representing the first date of endometriosis diagnosis, as the index date, 36 months of medical history was extracted for each patient. Historical data presented all available medical events in the patients' healthcare history before the condition diagnosis, including diagnoses for comorbid conditions, medical and surgical procedures, therapeutics, healthcare provider's specialty, and treatments prescribed to patients. A transactional level dataset, representing the top 1000 diagnosis codes, top 800 medical and surgical procedures, and top 500 prescribed drugs, was utilized to enable additional insights since these top codes constituted more than 80% of the dataset [21].

A pivot table was built at the transaction level and aggregated at the patient-level. Each row of the dataset represented an individual patient and the values within the row represented the counts of transactions that were generated during the patient's journey for the respective medical events. The columns of the table were the medical events, such as diagnosis and procedure codes, drugs prescribed, and physician specialties. The aggregated data table had more than 6 million rows and 2600 columns. The aggregated data table had missing values for selected patients and data elements, as not all records had complete medical information captured in the study period. Any medical events absent in the patient's history were represented with the value of *zero (0)*, which implied that no such event was observed in the individual's medical history. The final aggregated dataset was leveraged as an analytical dataset for the remaining parts of the chapter [21].

The analytical dataset was further normalized and divided into two groups: a training and test set. A ratio of 70:30 was applied to the dataset [28]. The training dataset was employed to identify the key data elements driving endometriosis diagnoses, while the test group was used to confirm whether these elements would predict the condition occurrence accurately [29]. Splitting the data into training and test sets aided the assessment of the model performance and its ability to generalize the hidden data trends [21, 30].

2.4 Overview of machine learning algorithms

In this section of the chapter, a summary of the classical statistical modeling and ML approaches is presented to review the available methods for healthcare research, and also to summarize the selected methodology applied in this study. Statistical modeling has evolved in the last few decades and shaped the future of business analytics and data science, including the current use and applications of ML algorithms [31]. It represents a branch of applied mathematics, in which statistical methods are leveraged to analyze a dataset. Statistical models are the mathematical representation of real-world scenarios with certain assumptions undertaken. They play a fundamental role in making statistical inferences while studying the characteristics of a population, upon which hypotheses were framed [8]. These models are not only useful in finding relationships between variables and the significance of those relationships, but they are also useful in the prediction and forecasting of future events.

ML is a subfield of the AI area, which includes statistics, mathematics, computer algorithms, etc., focused on building applications that learn and improve their predictive capabilities automatically over time without being specifically programmed to do so. ML models are built upon a statistical framework since they involve a large amount of data elements often described using statistical distributions. In the last two decades, ML algorithms have received a significant amount of attention in the fields of computer vision, natural language processing, autonomous driving vehicles, healthcare and drug development, e-commerce, to list a few due to the increased amounts of data availability and significant advancements in the computing power. ML algorithms can be broadly categorized as supervised, unsupervised, and semi-supervised algorithms [5, 7, 32, 33].

2.4.1 Supervised learning algorithms

Supervised learning is a set of algorithms that learn from the input space (X) to the output space (Y), i.e. $Y = f(X)$ [34]. The major objective is to estimate the mapping function (f) to ensure that with an addition of a new data point (x), the outcome, (y), could be predicted [35]. Supervised learning algorithms are often applied to classification and prediction problems [32]. The following are the selected examples of supervised algorithms often employed in research studies: *logistic regression, decision trees (DTs), random forest (RF), extreme gradient boosting, support vector machines (SVMs), Naïve Bayes, adaptive boosting (AdaBoost), artificial neural network (ANN), etc.* [36].

2.4.2 Unsupervised learning algorithms

Different from the supervised learning algorithms, the unsupervised learning algorithms try to understand the hidden patterns within the input dataset (X) [37]. The algorithms learn and uncover the patterns without the researcher's assistance [38]. These algorithms are often leveraged to find the naturally occurring clusters, reduce data dimensions, detect anomalies, etc. *k-means clustering, principal component analysis (PCA), factor analysis (FA), singular value decomposition (SVD), apriori algorithm (association rule)* represent a few examples of these types of algorithms [36]. In some cases, a semi-supervised approach is used to enhance the model performance with the help of a small amount of labeled data [36].

Depending on the study objectives and the availability and granularity of data, algorithms are reviewed for analytical relevance, tested for performance, data type fit, and selected as optimal algorithms accordingly. For this chapter, LR and XGB models were chosen to develop a predictive algorithm for the endometriosis onset. LR estimated the odds of the condition occurrence for a given medical event [39], while XGB provided more flexibility in fine-tuning the hyper-parameters when compared to other tree-based algorithms [40].

2.4.3 Logistic regression

An LR is a statistical model as well as the simplest version of ML algorithms that uses a logistic function to model a binary dependent variable with two possible outcomes: '*0*' and '*1*' [39, 41, 42]. A *multinomial logistic regression* is also often considered for research studies with multiple outcomes. LR is applied in a variety of fields, including healthcare research and social sciences [43].

In regression modeling, analysis often involves interpreting the independent variables' coefficients. Regression coefficients describe the size and direction of the relationship between regressors (x) and the outcome variable (y). They explain the behavior of the dependent variable given a unit change in an independent variable while holding all other data elements constant. The magnitude and sign of the coefficients signify the resulting relationship with the dependent variable. Interpreting the LR's coefficients also includetheir interpretation, as well as the odds and odds ratios [41].

Odds exemplify the ratio of probabilities of two mutually exclusive events [41], at the same time the *odds ratio* represents the ratio of two different odds. The simplest way to calculate the *odds ratio* in the LR is to exponentiate the coefficient of a predictor [39]. As a result, if the *odds ratio* for the age variable in years is 1.25, then for each additional year, the probability of event/success increases by 25%. For categorical features, the interpretation of the *odds ratio* can be more meaningful than the interpretation of *odds* [41].

2.4.4 xExtreme gradient boosting

A gradient boosting is another ML algorithm, which is an ensemble of simple, weak, and unreliable predictors, mainly decision trees [40]. When multiple trees are grouped, they create a robust and reliable algorithm [44]. XGB starts by creating a first simple tree [45] and builds upon the weaker learners. Each iteration revises the previous tree until an optimal point is reached [46].

Feature importance is the value generated by tree-based models, including *decision trees, random forest, XGB*, etc. [40]. The measure signifies the importance of features in the model as well as how good the feature is at reducing the node impurity. Feature importance is also known as *'gini importance'* or *'mean decrease impurity,'* and is defined as the total decrease in node impurity averaged over trees in the ensemble [44]. It is calculated as: *weight, gain, and cover*, where *'weight'* represents the number of times a feature is observed in a tree, *'gain'* denotes the average gain of splits, and *'cover'* is defined as the average coverage of splits. Finally, *coverage* represents the number of samples impacted by the split [46].

2.4.5 Chi-Square test

The Chi-Square test is nonparametric [33], often employed to test the independence between the observed and expected frequencies of one or more data elements. It is known as the *'goodness of fit test'* [47]. In this chapter, the Chi-Square test was utilized to select the top significant features [48].

2.4.6 p-value

The p-value is the probability of an observed result, assuming that the null hypothesis is correct. The p-value is used to test if the null hypothesis can be rejected in favor of the alternative hypothesis. A lower p-value implies a stronger indication in support of the alternative hypothesis [23]. In this analysis, the significance level was set at 5% to aid the feature importance evaluation and statistical results' identification.

2.4.7 Classification metrics

The following classification metrics are often leveraged to validate the ML models' performance. A confusion matrix is generated from the predicted probability values with *0.5* as the classification threshold. Patients with probability values greater than or equal to *0.5* are classified as *1* and below 0.5 are classified as 0. Below is the list of metrics used in evaluating models performance [32, 43, 46, 49]:

Confusion matrix:

- *True positive (TP)*—Target patient correctly identified by the model as target patient
- *False positive (FP)*—Control patient misclassified by the model as target patient
- *True negative (TN)*—Control patient correctly classified by the model as a control patient
- *False negative (FN)*—Target patient misclassified by the model as a control patient

Model performance metrics:

- *Accuracy:* % of total patients correctly identified among total patients
- *Positive predictive value (PPV, Precision):* % of true target patients among total predicted target patients
- *True positive rate (TPR, Sensitivity, Recall, Hit Rate):* % of true target patients who were correctly identified among total target patients
- *False positive rate (FPR):* % of true control patients incorrectly identified among total control patients
- *Specificity:* % of those control who will have a negative target result
- *F1 score:* is the harmonic mean of precision and recall
- *AUC*: Area under the receiver operating characteristic (ROC) curve. To validate the trade-off between true positive rate and false-positive rate

In this chapter, the LR, being the simplest of all ML algorithms, was chosen as the base model. Both the LR and XGB models were trained on the analytical dataset defined in the earlier section of this chapter. The top 1000 features from each algorithm were selected to reduce the dataset dimension. As the next step, the Chi-Square test from the *scikit-learn* Python package was utilized to identify the top most significant features from the list of data elements employed in both models. Finally, algorithms were re-trained on the top significant features to identify the key data elements in predicting the endometriosis onset. All ML algorithms were trained on Python 3.5 using '*scikit-learn*' and '*xgboost*' libraries.

3. Results

3.1 Important features selection

Table 3 presents the ML model performance metrics of the initial run, where the objective was to select the top features and study whether the data captured was

Algorithms	Statistic	Train set	Test set
LR	Accuracy	96%	96%
	Sensitivity/TPR/recall	95%	95%
	Specificity/TNR	98%	97%
	Precision/PPV	98%	97%
	f1-Score	0.96	0.96
	AUC	0.96	0.96
XGB	Accuracy	90%	88%
	Sensitivity/TPR/recall	86%	84%
	Specificity/TNR	95%	93%
	Precision/PPV	95%	92%
	f1-Score	0.9	0.88
	AUC	0.9	0.88

Table 3.
Classification metrics of train and test sets for LR and XGB model.

reasonably proven in disease prediction. Algorithms were trained on 70% of the analytical dataset and were tested on the remaining 30%. Metrics captured indicated that both the LR and XGB models performed relatively well in predicting the condition onset. The models' accuracy ranged between 88% and 96%. **Figure 2** presents the ROC curves on the test set for LR and XGB models respectively. The area under the ROC curve (AUC) values were 0.88 and 0.96, respectively for both models.

From the outputs of the initial model run, the top 1000 features with absolute regressor coefficients in descending order greater than zero (*0*) were selected from the LR. Similarly, another set of top 1000 features with feature importance greater than zero (*0*) were identified from XGB. Both sets were combined to establish a unique list of top features. As the next step, the Chi-Square test for feature selection from Python *scikit-learn* package was applied to select the top 1000 most significant features for the final model run. The top features were selected at a standard significance level of 5% (α = 0.05). Most of the top significant features were associated with a series of medical and surgical procedures, as well as various diagnostic and comorbid conditions.

As noted above, **Table 4** presents the list of most significant features identified by the Chi-Square test, which were associated with the endometriosis diagnosis.

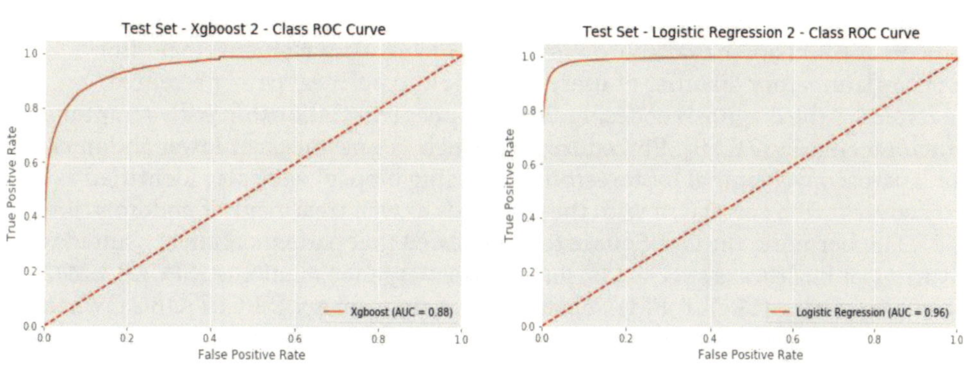

Figure 2.
XGB & LR ROC curves on test set.

Feature	Feature description	Chi–square	LR: feature coefficients
D N85_8	Other specified non-inflammatory disorder of uterus	0	3.48
D_N94_6	Dysmenorrhea, unspecifie	0	0.17
D_N94_9	Unspecified condition associated with female genital organs and menstrual cycle	0	6.9
D_R10_2	Pelvic and perineal pain	0	−0.04
D_Z01_419	Encounter for gynecological examination (general) (routine) without abnormal findings	0	−1.95
P_00840	Anesthesia intraperitoneal lower abd w/laps nos	0	1.54
P_00944	Anesthesia vaginal hysterectomy incl biopsy	0	1.55
P_52000	Cystourethroscopy	0	5.78
P_58571	Laps total hysterect 250 gm/<w/rmvl tube/ovary	0	3.25
P_58573	Laparoscopy tot hysterectomy >250 g w/tube/ovar	0	5.31
P_58662	Laps fulg/exc ovary viscera/ peritoneal surface	0	4.17
P_76830	Us transvaginal	0	1.93
P_J1950	Injection. Leuprolide acetate (for depot suspens)	0	3.74
R_Norethindrone_Acetate	Norethindrone acetate	0	0.26
SPCLT_EM	Emergency medicine	0	−9.47
SPCLT_FM	Family medicine	0	−3.63
SPCLT_HO	Hematology/oncology	0	−4.6
SPCLT_OBG	Obstetrics and gynecology	0	−2.43

Table 4.
Most significant features from LR, XGB, and Chi-Square test.

The table also presents the LR coefficients to provide relative direction between the endometriosis onset and the selected top regressors. As noted in the earlier version of the chapter available on Research Square, data elements including 'non-inflammatory disorder of uterus,' 'pelvic and perineal pain' presented examples of the diagnosis codes, indicated a positive relationship with symptoms of endometriosis [21, 50]. Procedure codes such as 'anesthesia of lower abdomen for laparoscopy,' 'vaginal hysterectomy including biopsy' were also identified as the procedures often correlated with the diagnosis as well treatment of endometriosis [50]. Furthermore, the Chi-Square test suggested that patients often consulted with a variety of healthcare specialists, including 'emergency medicine (SPCLT_EM),' 'family medicine (SPCLT_FM),' 'obstetrics and gynecology (SPCLT_OBG)' when experiencing gynecological symptoms and concerns; however, a larger number of office visits might negatively impact the likelihood for the condition diagnosis, as noted by the negative regressor coefficients.

3.2 Feature selection for the cohort selection

The significant features from Section 3.1, which were specific to the target cohort, seemed promising in defining the drivers of the endometriosis condition onset, and hence, were selected to identify the patient base list for scorning. Therapeutics as well as medical and surgical procedure codes specific to endometriosis treatment such as Orilissa, Marilissa, and Lupron Depot, were excluded from the analysis to avoid introducing any biases into the next phase of the study. Around 9.5 million female patients age 18 and above qualified for the scoring process.

3.3 Machine learning model training and outcome validation

The LR and XGB models were re-trained, using the top significant features. A drop in the model performance at the beginning of the re-training process was observed. After several iterations and hyper-parameter tuning, the predictive power of the XGB model significantly improved compared to the previous iterations; however, no improvement in the LR model performance metrics was observed. Interestingly, both models were able to identify additional new features aligned with endometriosis.

Table 5 presents the top features identified by the XGB and LR models to be important in predicting the likelihood of endometriosis along with the statistical measures and metrics to assess the importance and significance of the features. The Chi-Square test (p-value) signified the importance of data elements in differentiating the target and control patients. The XGB feature importance weighed the value of features in the model in predicting the outcome. Similarly, the LR odds ratios helped to understand the odds of being diagnosed with endometriosis, given a particular medical event.

Overall, results suggest that features including 'other ovarian cyst, right side,' 'hypertrophy of uterus,' 'submucous leiomyoma of uterus,' 'excessive bleeding in the premenopausal period,' 'unspecified condition associated with female genital organs,' and 'menstrual cycle' were important in predicting the likelihood of endometriosis. The models had also flagged 'acetaminophen' and 'megestrol acetate' drugs as strong predictors of the condition.

Table 6 shows that the XGB model performed better overall compared to the LR model. **Figure 3** shows the receiver operating characteristic (ROC) curves on the test sets for both re-trained models. The area under the ROC curve (AUC) values of the LR and XGB models were 0.87 and 0.96, respectively. Furthermore, **Figure 4** suggests that the XGB model was able to differentiate more accurately the targets from the controls than the LR model; hence, based on the final model results, the XGB model was utilized to score the qualified patients.

3.4 Scoring qualified patients

The last step of the model evaluation was to score the qualified patients to assess the model's accuracy in predicting the endometriosis onset. A sample of 9.5 million patients was identified and complete medical history was extracted for 36 months. After dataset preparation, the probability of endometriosis was estimated, leveraging the re-trained XGB model.

Probability distribution of 9.5 million scored patients is shown in **Figure 5**. Most of the predicted probability values were concentrated either toward '*0*' or '*1*'. When considering *0.5* as a threshold, the XGB model identified around 36% of the scored patients as being likely to receive an endometriosis diagnosis within the next

Feature	Long description	Chi-square (p)	XGB_feature_ importance	LR_beta_ coeff	Odds_ratio
P_58662	Laps fulg/exc ovary viscera/peritoneal surface	0	0.0318	4.70	109.73
P_58571	Laps total hysterect 250 gm/< w/rmvl tube/ovary	0	0.0212	4.17	64.53
D_N85_8	Other specified noninflammatory disorders of uterus	0	0.0094	2.56	12.88
D_N83_291	Other ovarian cyst, right side	0	0.0092	2.84	17.06
P_58661	Laparoscopy w/rmvl adnexal structures	0	0.0089	2.43	11.32
D_N85_2	Hypertrophy of uterus	0	0.0088	2.67	14.42
P_00944	Anesthesia vaginal hysterectomy incl biopsy	0	0.0076	1.77	5.86
P_52000	Cystourethroscopy	0	0.0075	1.62	5.04
D_D25_2	Subserosal leiomyoma of uterus	0	0.0069	2.25	9.53
P_72197	mri pelvis w/o & w/contrast material	0	0.0067	2.72	15.17
R_ACETAMINOPHEN	Acetaminophen	0	0.0066	2.01	7.46
D_N81_4	Uterovaginal prolapse, unspecified	0	0.0063	1.86	6.40
D_N94_9	Unspecified condition associated with female genital organs and menstrual cycle	0	0.0063	2.57	13.10
D_N92_4	Excessive bleeding in the premenopausal period	0	0.0061	2.30	9.99
D_D25_0	Submucous leiomyoma of uterus	0	0.0059	2.46	11.76
D_R10_2	Pelvic and perineal pain	0	0.0056	0.60	1.83
D_N94_5	Secondary dysmenorrheal	0	0.0056	2.81	16.64
D_Z79_890	Hormone replacement therapy	0	0.0047	2.23	9.34
D_Z80_41	Family history of malignant neoplasm of ovary	0	0.0045	2.12	8.37
D_N94_3	Premenstrual tension syndrome	0	0.0042	2.43	11.37
R_LIDOCAINE_HCL	Lidocaine hcl	0	0.0041	2.12	8.30

Feature	Long description	Chi-square (p)	XGB_feature_importance	LR_beta_coeff	Odds_ratio
R_MEGESTROL_ACETATE	Megestrol acetate	0	0.0039	2.19	8.94
D_F43_0	Acute stress reaction	0	0.0032	2.36	10.61
D_N94_12	Deep dyspareunia	0	0.0023	2.35	10.51
D_N97_0	Female infertility associated with anovulation	0	0.0022	2.19	8.89
SPCLT_AN	Anesthesiology	0	0.0012	(0.55)	0.58
SPCLT_DR	Diagnostic radiology	0	0.0009	(0.87)	0.42
SPCLT_OBG	Obstetrics and gynecology	0	0.0008	(0.64)	0.53
SPCLT_EM	Emergency medicine	0	0.0006	(1.92)	0.15
SPCLT_FM	Family medicine	0	0.0004	(1.05)	0.35
SPCLT_IM	Internal medicine	0	0.0004	(0.92)	0.40
SPCLT_HO	Hematology/oncology	0	0.0003	(0.79)	0.45

Table 5.
List of top features identified by the re-trained models.

Algorithms	Statistic	Train set	Test set
LR	Accuracy	87%	87%
	Sensitivity/TPR/recall	75%	75%
	Specificity/TNR	98%	98%
	Precision/PPV	98%	98%
	f1-score	0.85	0.85
	AUC	0.87	0.87
XGB	Accuracy	96%	94%
	Sensitivity/TPR/recall	93%	90%
	Specificity/TNR	99%	98%
	Precision/PPV	99%	97%
	f1-score	0.96	0.93
	AUC	0.96	0.94

Table 6.
Classification metric of LR and XGB model on train and test set.

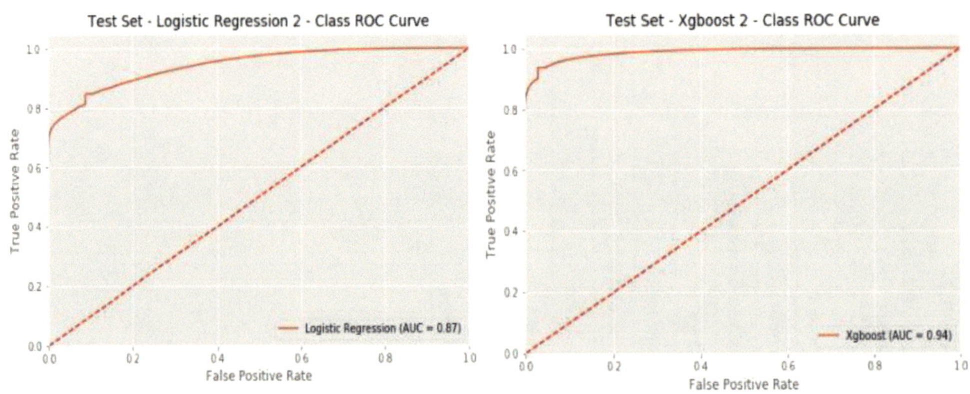

Figure 3.
ROC curves of LR and XG models on test set.

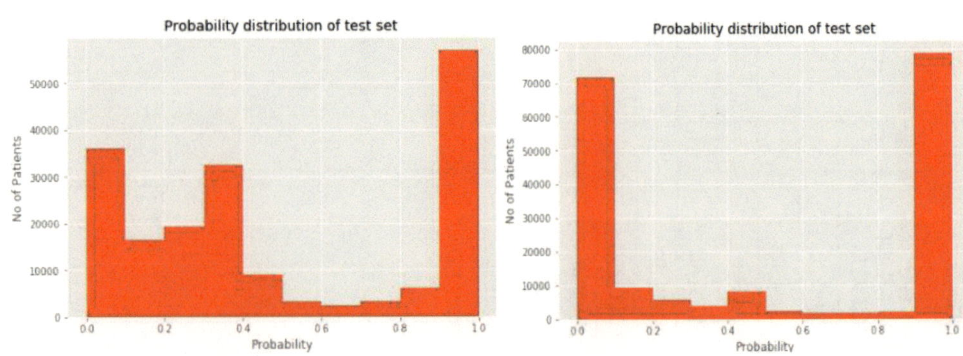

Figure 4.
Distribution of probability on test data set for both the LR and XGB models. Figure on right side is of XGB and most of scores are grouped at extreme values.

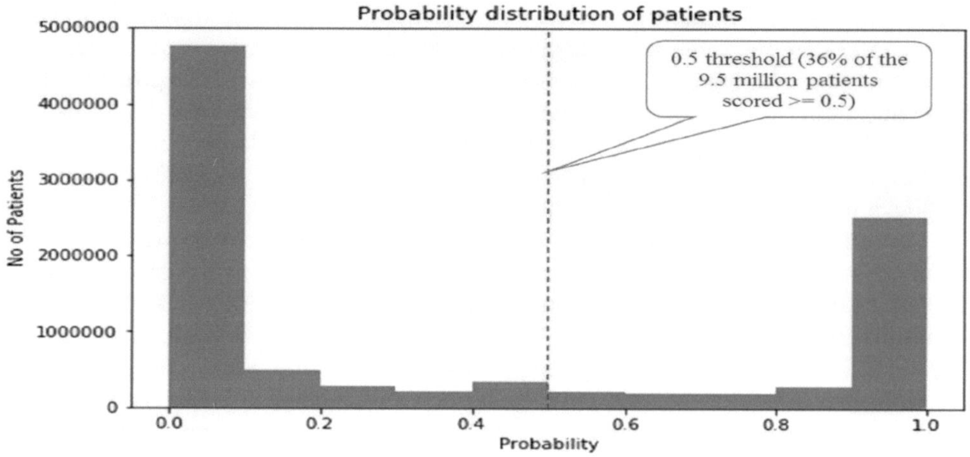

Figure 5.
Distribution of patients by predicted probability score.

12 months. Assuming an ability to leverage the significant variables in diagnosing the condition onset, practitioners could provide focused and specialized medical care in time to their patients, thereby, reducing the risks of endometriosis and its related complications.

There is also a different way to present the data elements driving the prediction of disease onset and the scoring of patients for the likelihood of the disease. A nomogram (otherwise known as nomograph) is defined as an alignment chart or a two-dimensional diagram applied to estimate the graphical computation of a mathematical function [51]. A nomogram comprises a set of scales, where each scale denotes a selected feature of the studied population.

The nomogram tool is often employed in clinical medicine to predict patients' outcomes when considering their clinical features [52]. It is also used in clinical oncology to aid healthcare providers in their treatment decisions. It leverages regression models

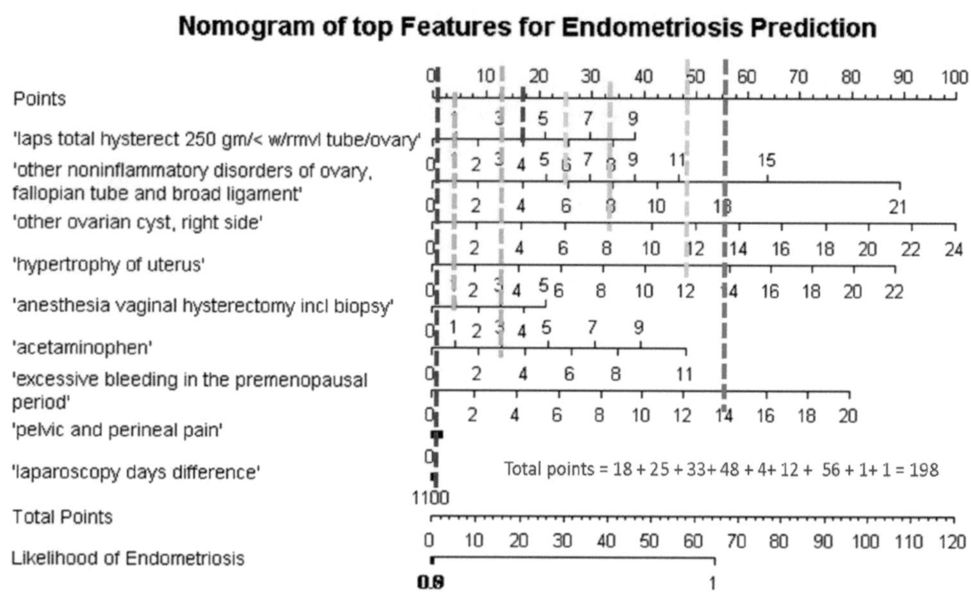

Figure 6.
Nomogram of top features to predict likelihood of endometriosis.

such as the LR and parametric survival model as the basis for its framework [53]. For this chapter, a nomogram was selected to present a selected group of top features important to predicting the likelihood of endometriosis, as shown in **Figure 6**. The following attributes were noted on the chart as important in driving the diagnosis: 'laps total hysterect 250 gm/< w/rmvl tube/ovary,' 'other noninflammatory disorders of ovary, fallopian tube, and broad ligament,' 'other ovarian cyst, right side,' 'hypertrophy of uterus,' 'acetaminophen,' and 'pelvic and perineal pain.'

To predict the disease onset, the contribution of each feature was measured as a point score (topmost axis in the nomogram) based on the values that each feature could take with individual point scores being added to determine the likelihood of endometriosis onset. When the value of the feature was '*0*', its contribution was '*0*'points. The dotted line depicted the point score for an individual value of each respective feature with the total point being *198*, which implied a very high probability of the disease onset. Nomogram was found to be a helpful tool to graphically study the outcomes given a group of few features; however, it was also challenging to leverage it, knowing a large number of studied features [52, 53].

4. Discussion

As mentioned in Section 3, the LR and XGB ML models were able to identify the top features that could help to explain endometriosis onset in advance. **Tables 4** and **5** present the important features to predict the condition onset. These features included diagnosis codes, medical and surgical procedure codes, as well as physician specialties that often support patients through their healthcare journey.

Furthermore, **Table 5** also presents the *LR odds ratio* and XGB feature importance index to aid the understanding and interpretation of the results. As noted in the above section, *odds ratios* defined the odds of being diagnosed with endometriosis when the feature changes by a unit, holding other features constant. For example, the *odds ratio* of 'uterovaginal prolapse, unspecified' was 6.40, which implied that for every additional diagnosis of 'uterovaginal prolapse, unspecified', the odds of endometriosis went up by 540%. Similarly, if a patient had an additional appointment with an 'obstetrics and gynecology' specialist then the odds decreased by 47%.

As a reminder, the first part of the ML analysis was to identify the top features from an extensive list of data elements (**Table 4**). LR, XGB, and Chi-Square tests were employed to derive the final list of features to re-train the model. **Table 5** presents the most promising features with their respective significance and importance values. A number of the variables from the model were also cited in other medical and scientific journal publications, including articles from Johns Hopkins Medicine [17] and Queensland Health [18] on endometriosis signs, symptoms, and diagnosis, which confirmed the model's validity from the medical and clinical side.

In the next part of this section, the selected most important features by their respective groups were reviewed and evaluated for their relevance to the endometriosis diagnostic process. The preliminary insights for this research are available on the Research Square website. The advanced preview allowed for valuable feedback that helped to enhance the research design for this chapter.

1. Diagnoses codes: 'other ovarian cyst, right side', 'unspecified condition associated with female genital organs and menstrual cycle,' 'other specified noninflammatory disorders of the uterus,' 'excessive bleeding in the premenopausal period,' 'female pelvic peritoneal adhesions (post-infective),' 'uterovaginal prolapse, unspecified', etc. clearly showed association with the risks and symptoms

of endometriosis [54]. Feature importance from XGB suggested that these features drove the model, whereas *odds ratio* from LR also indicated the direction of increase or decrease in odds of getting diagnosed with the condition. To further define the magnitude of importance, **Table 5** presents that if a patient was diagnosed with 'excessive bleeding in the premenopausal period' then the odds of receiving endometriosis diagnosis in the near future increased by 899%. Similar to these findings, Mayo Clinic articles also stated that patients might experience occasional heavy bleeding before being diagnosed with the condition [55].

2. Medical and surgical procedures: 'laps fulg/exc ovary viscera/peritoneal surface', 'laps total hysterect 250 gm/< w/rmvl tube/ovary', 'anesthesia vaginal hysterectomy incl biopsy', 'laparoscopy w/rmvl adnexal structures', 'MRI pelvis w/o & w/contrast material,' 'cystourethroscopy', etc. were also associated with the diagnosis as well treatment of endometriosis. The finding showed that for every additional procedure on 'mri of pelvis,' the odds of endometriosis increased by 1471%. Recent research from Abdominal Radiology, published by Springer Nature, also supported this claim that MRI could be more precise in the diagnosis of endometriosis compared to other diagnostic techniques [56].

As presented in **Table 5**, the procedure 'laps total hysterect 250 gm/< w/rmvl tube/ovary' had the odds ratio of 64.53, which implied that if a patient had a 'laparoscopy with hysterectomy' then the odds of endometriosis onset increased significantly. Previous studies on endometriosis also cited 'laparoscopy procedure as the gold standard' in the diagnosis process [8]. However, while the nomogram graph (**Figure 6**) also suggested that a patient was likely to get diagnosed with endometriosis post this procedure, the data element was further analyzed to understand how it might have correlated to the actual diagnoses, knowing that many laparoscopic procedures were performed to treat other female gynecological conditions. **Figure 6** shows that the feature 'laparoscope days difference' presented little importance in predicting the likelihood of the disease onset. The data element measured the significance of laparoscopic procedures in predicting the likelihood of endometriosis via calculating the days' difference between the laparoscopic procedure and the event date for both target and control cohorts.

Furthermore, the additional analysis revealed that around 60% of the target patients compared to only about 5% of the control group were diagnosed with endometriosis after a laparoscopic procedure performed on the same day of diagnosis. This finding implies that laparoscopy might not actually be a significant driver of the endometriosis diagnosis as presented in the XGB model when accounting for the time component before the diagnosis, although there were statistical significant differences between the two groups.

3. From the patient medical journey and healthcare access side, the ML models suggested that patients often consult with multiple healthcare specialists, including 'emergency medicine,' 'family medicine,' 'hematology/oncology,' 'internal medicine,' 'obstetrics and gynecology' when experiencing endometriosis-related symptoms and gynecological issues. Since, endometriosis tends to be difficult to diagnose, patients often had a number of unrelated office visits with symptoms associated later with endometriosis. This finding presented that many female patients faced substantial challenges in receiving proper care and treatment. Consequently, patients visited multiple specialists in search of answers for their signs and symptoms [57]. In agreement with these statements, both LR and XGB models presented negative weights and low importance to these healthcare providers' features, which suggested that if

a patient visited these specialists more frequently, the longer it took to receive a confirmatory endometriosis diagnosis.

Furthermore, women with a history of endometriosis were found more likely to be diagnosed with either an 'ovarian cancer' or 'endometriosis-associated adenocarcinoma' in the future [21, 58–60]. With this in mind, having the ML models identify 'hematology/oncology (SPCLT_HO),' as one of the top Board Certified specialties, further suggested that an office visit with an oncologist should be recommended for any patients presenting signs and symptoms as noted above to rule out any potential cancer risk [21, 61, 62].

4. LR and XGB models also identified additional data elements, which were important in predicting the likelihood of endometriosis onset. The models suggested, as noted in the earlier version of the chapter posted on the Research Square website that data elements like 'deep dyspareunia,' 'female infertility associated with anovulation,' 'premenstrual tension syndrome,' 'hormone replacement therapy,' 'family history of malignant neoplasm of ovary' were identified as highly significant to the prediction endometriosis. Past medical articles supported these claims of fibroids, ovarian cysts, infertility, menstrual period complications, family history of neoplasm of the ovary, hormone therapy, etc. having a strong association with the condition [21, 54]. Furthermore, the finding that women of reproductive age who experience chronic stress were also at a higher risk of developing endometriosis was noted in other medical articles, implying that healthcare providers should consider this symptom in their diagnostic process [21, 63].

5. As mentioned in the preliminary version of the chapter on the Research Square website, 'acetaminophen,' 'megestrol acetate,' 'lidocaine hcl,' etc. were found to be strong predictors of endometriosis occurrence, as these drugs were often prescribed as analgesics to help control pelvic pain. Data elements, including 'submucous leiomyoma of the uterus' and 'hypertrophy of uterus,' were identified as the significant predictors as well [55, 64]; however, more clinical research is required in support of this claim, as these diseases presented similar symptoms, which might impact the ability for healthcare providers to diagnose endometriosis [21, 65].

Overall, the analysis results presented the important data elements to be considered when diagnosing endometriosis in women of reproductive age, to time more accurately disease onset and aid the diagnostic process. As noted in Section 3, when leveraging these features in the diagnostic process, a high accuracy prediction of the disease occurrence was identified, with the model differentiating with high precision between patients with and without the condition. Furthermore, a nomogram graphical representation could be leveraged as one of the tools to graphically predict the outcome given a set of features. Top features were utilized to showcase the practicality of the tool; however, the tool has limitations on the number of data elements that could be applied in the analysis.

5. Conclusions

In this chapter, the crucial role of AI and ML algorithms in disease diagnosis prediction and forecasting was presented, studied, and validated. Patient medical history was leveraged for the ML analysis. LR and XGB models identified important medical attributes, which were then leveraged to predict the likelihood of endometriosis onset. Early diagnosis can offer an opportunity for women to receive required medical care much earlier in the patient journey.

Leveraging the findings of this study and other related studies can help inform the development of analytical tools and algorithms to be integrated into the Electronic Health Records (EHR) systems to simplify and enhance the diagnosing activities performed by healthcare providers. The enhancements could further inform the diagnostic processes to aid in a timely and precise diagnostic process, ultimately increasing the quality of patient care and life.

Future research should focus on enhancing the ML analysis and exploring advanced deep learning methodologies to improve the accuracy and precision of the current results. Furthermore, imputing the missing data elements with mean and mode values, or even predictive models, can further augment the model performance and increase the accuracy of the ML models in predicting the likelihood of the disease onset. Creating time-based variables (30, 60, 120 days before diagnosis) to account for the time to endometriosis diagnosis would add a significant improvement in the feature engineering step to help with establishing a timeline of events important in the endometriosis diagnostic process.

Acknowledgements

Authors would like to recognize Heather Valera, Suzanne Rosado, and Koichi Iwata for their review of document drafts, and their valuable feedback in improving the article content.

Funding

Authors work for Symphony Health, ICON plc Organization. The data used in the article is the property of Symphony Health, ICON plc Organization. Authors used the healthcare claims data for the sole purpose of publication of this article.

Competing interest

The authors declare that they have no competing interests.

Availability of data and materials

The dataset leveraged for this chapter is a property of Symphony Health, ICON, plc. Data sharing restrictions apply to the availability of these data, and therefore, the dataset is not available for public use.

Author details

Ewa J. Kleczyk[1*], Tarachand Yadav[2] and Stalin Amirtharaj[2]

1 Symphony Health, ICON, plc, Blue Bell, PA, USA

2 ICON, plc, Blue Bell, PA, USA

*Address all correspondence to: ewa.kleczyk@symphonyhealth.com

References

[1] Doupe P, Faghmous J, Basu S. Machine learning for health services researchers. Value Health. 2019;**22**(7):808-815. Available from: https://pubmed.ncbi.nlm.nih.gov/31277828/ [Accessed: October 1, 2020]

[2] Crown WH. Potential application of machine learning in health outcomes research and some statistical cautions. International Society for Pharmacoeconomics and Outcomes Research (ISPOR). 2015. DOI: 10.1016/j.jval.2014.12.005 [Accessed: October 1, 2020]

[3] Ghassemi M, Naumann T, Schulam P, Beam AL, Chen IY, Ranganath R. A review of challenges and opportunities in machine learning for health. arXivLabs. 2019. Available from: https://arxiv.org/abs/1806.00388 [Accessed: October 1, 2020]

[4] Buch VH, Ahmed I, Maruthappu M. Artificial intelligence in medicine: Current trends and future possibilities. British Journal of General Practice. 2018;**68**(668):143-144. DOI: 10.3399/bjgp18X695213 [Accessed: October 1, 2020]

[5] Rajkomar A, Lingam S, Taylor AG, Blum M, Mongan J. High-throughput classification of radiographs using deep convolutional neural networks. Journal of Digital Imaging. 2016;**30**:95-101. DOI: 10.1007/s10278-016-9914-9

[6] Chen M, Hao Y, Hwang K, Wang L, Wang L. Disease prediction by machine learning over big data from healthcare communities. IEEE. 2017;**5**:8869-8879. DOI: 10.1109/ACCESS.2017.2694446 [Accessed: October 1, 2020]

[7] Alexandru AG, Radu IM, Bizon ML. Big data in healthcare—Opportunities and challenges. Informatica Economică. 2018;**22**(2):43-54. DOI: 10.12948/issn14531305/22.2.2018.05

[8] Rolla E. Endometriosis: Advances and controversies in classification, pathogenesis, diagnosis, and treatment. Version 1. F1000Research. 2019;**8**:F1000. DOI: 10.12688/f1000research.14817.1. Available from: https://www.ncbi.nlm.nih.gov/pmc/articles/PMC6480968/ [Accessed: March 30, 2021]

[9] Chapron C, Fauconnier A, Goffinet F, Breart G, Dubuisson JB. Laparoscopic surgery is not inherently dangerous for patients presenting with benign gynaecologic pathology. Results of a meta-analysis. Human Reproduction. 2002;**17**:1334-1342

[10] Parasar P, Ozcan P, Terry KL. Endometriosis: Epidemiology, diagnosis and clinical management. Current Obstetrics and Gynecology Reports. 2017;**6**(1):34-41. DOI: 10.1007/s13669-017-0187-1

[11] Hoogeveen M, Dorr PJ, Puylaert JBCM. Endometriosis of the rectovaginal septum: Endovaginal US and MRI findings in two cases. Abdominal Imaging. 2003;**28**:897-901

[12] Akter S, Xu D, Nagel SC, Bromfield JJ, Pelch KE, Wilshire GB, et al. GenomeForest: An ensemble machine learning classifier for endometriosis. AMIA Joint Summits on Translational Science proceedings. 2020;**2020**:33-42

[13] Sadia A, Dong X, Nagel Susan C, Bromfield John J, Katherine P, Wilshire Gilbert B, et al. Machine learning classifiers for endometriosis using transcriptomics and methylomics data. Frontiers in Genetics. 2019;**10**:766. DOI: 10.3389/fgene.2019.00766

[14] Nnoaham KE, Hummelshoj L, Kennedy SH, Jenkinson C, Zondervan KT, World Endometriosis Research Foundation Women's Health

Symptom Survey Consortium. Developing symptom-based predictive models of endometriosis as a clinical screening tool: Results from a multicenter study. Fertility and Sterility. 2012;**98**(3):692-701.e5. DOI: 10.1016/j.fertnstert.2012.04.022. Epub 2012 May 30

[15] Noventa M, Saccardi C, Litta P, Vitagliano A, D'Antona D, Abdulrahim B, et al. Ultrasound techniques in the diagnosis of deep pelvic endometriosis: Algorithm based on a systematic review and meta-analysis. Fertility and Sterility. 2015;**104**(2):366-383.e2. DOI: 10.1016/j.fertnstert.2015.05.002

[16] Zhang Y, Wang Z, Zhang J, et al. Deep learning model for classifying endometrial lesions. Journal of Translational Medicine. 2021;**19**:10. DOI: 10.1186/s12967-020-02660-x

[17] Endometriosis signs and symptoms. Available from: https://www.hopkinsmedicine.org/health/conditions-and-diseases/endometriosis [Accessed: October 1, 2020]

[18] Endometriosis signs and symptoms. Available from: https://www.health.qld.gov.au/news-events/news/signs-symptoms-endometriosis [Accessed: October 1, 2020]

[19] PRA Health Sciences. Data Insights. Available from: https://prahs.com/healthcare-intelligence/data-insights

[20] Symphony Health Solutions. Available from: https://symphonyhealth.prahs.com/

[21] Kleczyk EJ, Peri A, Yadav T, Komera R, Peri M, Guduru V, et al. Prsedicting endometriosis onset using machine learning algorithms. ResearchSquare. Available from: https://www.researchsquare.com/article/rs-135736/v1. 10.21203/rs.3.rs-135736/v1 [Accessed: October 4, 2021]

[22] Getting the Most Out of Longitudinal Patient Data. Anonymous patient-level data (APLD). Available from: https://www.rxdatascience.com/blog/getting-most-out-of-longitudinal-patient-data [Accessed: October 1, 2020]

[23] Marketing, Patient Data, and Privacy Concerns. Available from: https://www.reutersevents.com/pharma/commercial/marketing-patient-data-and-privacy-concerns [Accessed: October 5, 2020]

[24] Integrated Dataverse (IDV®). https://symphonyhealth.prahs.com/what-we-do/view-health-data [Accessed: October 1, 2020]

[25] Symphony Health Solutions, What We Do. Available from: https://symphonyhealth.prahs.com/what-we-do

[26] Ali MS, Prieto-Alhambra D, Lopes C, Ramos D, Bispo N, Ichihara MY, et al. Propensity score methods in health technology assessment: Principles, extended applications, and recent advances. Frontiers in Pharmacology. 2019;**10**:973. DOI: 10.3389/fphar.2019.00973 [Accessed: October 1, 2020]

[27] Rosenbaum PR, Rubin DB. The central role of the propensity score in observational studies for causal effects. Biometrika. 1983;**70**:41-55. DOI: 10.1093/biomet/70.1.41 [Accessed: October 1, 2020]

[28] Rosenbaum PR, Rubin DB. Constructing a control group using multivariate matched sampling methods that incorporate the propensity score. The American Statistician. 1985;**39**(1):33-38. DOI: 10.1080/00031305.1985.10479383 [Accessed: October 1, 2020]

[29] Xu Y, Goodacre R. On splitting training and validation set: A comparative study of cross-validation,

bootstrap and systematic sampling for estimating the generalization performance of supervised learning. Journal of Analysis and Testing. 2017;**2**(3):249-262. DOI: 10.1007/s41664-018-0068-2 [Accessed: October 1, 2020]

[30] Ballantyne Draelos RL. Best Use of Train/Val/Test Splits, with Tips for Medical Data. Glass Box Machine Learning and Medicine. Available from: https://glassboxmedicine.com/2019/09/15/best-use-of-train-val-test-splits-with-tips-for-medical-data/. [Accessed: October 5, 2020]

[31] Bzdok D, Altman N, Krzywinski M. Statistics versus machine learning. Nature Methods. 2018;**15**:233-234. DOI: 10.1038/nmeth.4642 [Accessed: March 30, 2021]

[32] Simeone O. A very brief introduction to machine learning with applications to communication systems. arXiv preprint arXiv:1808.02342v4. 2018

[33] Cochran WG. The Chi-square test of goodness of fit. The Annals of Mathematical Statistics. 1952;**23**(3):315-345. DOI: 10.1214/aoms/1177729380 [Accessed: October 5, 2020

[34] Vabalas A, Gowen E, Poliakoff E, Casson AJ. Machine learning algorithm validation with a limited sample size. Plos One. 2019;**14**(11):20. DOI: 10.1371/journal.pone.0224365 [Accessed: October 5, 2020]

[35] Kotsiantis SB. Supervised machine learning: A review of classification techniques. Informatica. 2007;**31**:249-268

[36] Hinton G, Sejnowski T. Unsupervised Learning: Foundations of Neural Computation. Cambridge, MA: MIT Press; 1999. pp. vii-xv. ISBN: 978-0262581684

[37] Wosiak A, Zamecznik A, Niewiadomska-Jarosik K. Supervised and unsupervised machine learning for improved identification of intrauterine growth restriction types. In: Federated Conference on Computer Science and Information Systems (FedCSIS). Gdańsk, Poland: IEEE; 2016

[38] Hastie T, Tibshirani R, Friedman J. "Unsupervised Learning," The Elements of Statistical Learning. New York, NY: Springer Series in Statistics, Springer; 2009. pp. 485-585

[39] Logistic Regression. Available from: https://en.wikipedia.org/wiki/Logistic_regression

[40] Friedman JH. Greedy function approximation: A gradient boosting machine. The Annals of Statistics. 2001;**29**:1189-1232. DOI: 10.1214/aos/1013203451 [Accessed: October 1, 2020]

[41] Cramer JS. The origins of logistic regression. Tinbergen Institute Discussion Paper. TI 2002-119/4. Available from: https://papers.tinbergen.nl/02119.pdf [Accessed: October 1, 2020]

[42] Hosmer DW, Lemeshow S. Applied Logistic Regression. New York: Wiley; 2013. ISBN: 978-0-470-58247-3

[43] Agresti A. Categorical Data Analysis. Hoboken: John Wiley and Sons; 2012. ISBN: 978-0-470-46363-5

[44] Extreme Gradient Boosting. Available from: https://xgboost.readthedocs.io/en/latest/tutorials/model.html

[45] Chen T, Guestrin C. XGBoost: A scalable tree boosting system. In: Krishnapuram B, Shah M, Smola AJ, Aggarwal CC, Shen D, Rastogi R, editors. Proceedings of the 22nd ACM SIGKDD International Conference on Knowledge Discovery and Data Mining; August 13-17, 2016; San Francisco, CA, USA. ACM; 2016. pp. 785-794.

DOI: 10.1145/2939672.2939785 [Accessed: October 5, 2020]

[46] Hastie T, Tibshirani R, Friedman JH. '10. Boosting and Additive Trees'. The Elements of Statistical Learning. 2nd ed. New York: Springer; 2009. pp. 337-384

[47] On the interpretation of χ2 from contingency tables, and the calculation of p. Journal of the Royal Statistical Society. 1922;**85**(1):87-94. DOI: 10.2307/2340521

[48] Chi-Square feature selection. "Scikit-learn" Python Library. Available from: https://scikit-learn.org/stable/modules/generated/sklearn.feature_selection.chi2.html [Accessed: October 5, 2020]

[49] Manning CD, Raghavan P, Schütze H. Introduction to Information Retrieval. Feature Selection, Chi-Square Feature Selection. Cambridge, UK: Cambridge University Press; 2008

[50] OBG Management. Endometriosis and infertility: Expert answers to 6 questions to help pinpoint the best route to pregnancy. Mdedge ObGyn. 2015;**27**(6):30-35. Available from: https://www.mdedge.com/obgyn/article/99912/surgery/endometriosis-and-infertility-expert-answers-6-questions-help-pinpoint/ [Accessed: October 5, 2020]

[51] Kattan MW, Marasco J. What is a real nomogram? Seminars in Oncology. 2010;**37**:23-26

[52] Su D, Zhou X, Chen Q, et al. Prognostic nomogram for thoracic esophageal squamous cell carcinoma after radical esophagectomy. PLoS One. 2015;**10**:e0124437

[53] Breiman L. Statistical modeling: The two cultures (with comments and a rejoinder by the author). Statistical Science. 2001;**16**(3):199-231. DOI: 10.1214/ss/1009213726 [Accessed: March 30, 2021]

[54] Endometriosis—Risks, Signs, Symptoms, Diagnosis and Treatment. Available from: https://www.mayoclinic.org/diseases-conditions/endometriosis/symptoms-causes/syc-20354656 [Accessed: October 5, 2020]

[55] Liang B, Xie YG, Xu XP, Hu CH. Diagnosis and treatment of submucous myoma of the uterus with interventional ultrasound. Oncology Letters. 2018;**15**(5):6189-6194. DOI: 10.3892/ol.2018.8122 [Accessed: October 5, 2020]

[56] Tong A, VanBuren WM, Chamié L, Feldman M, Hindman N, Huang C, et al. Recommendations for MRI Technique in the evaluation of pelvic endometriosis: Consensus statement from the Society of Abdominal Radiology Endometriosis Disease-Focused Panel. Abdominal Radiology. 2020;**45**(6):1569-1586. DOI: 10.1007/s00261-020-02483-w [Accessed: March 30, 2021]

[57] Agarwal SK, Antunez-Flores O, Foster WG, et al. Real-world characteristics of women with endometriosis-related pain entering a multidisciplinary endometriosis program. BMC Women's Health. 2021;**21**:19. DOI: 10.1186/s12905-020-01139-7 [Accessed: March 30, 2021]

[58] Kvaskoff M, Horne AW, Missmer SA. Informing women with endometriosis about ovarian cancer risk. The Lancet Journal. 2017;**390**(10111):2433-2434. DOI: 10.1016/S0140-6736(17)33049-0 [Accessed: October 5, 2020]

[59] Brilhante A, Augusto KL, Cavalcante Portela M, Sucupira L, Oliveira F, Pouchaim A, et al. Endometriosis and ovarian cancer: An integrative review (endometriosis and ovarian cancer). Asian Pacific Journal of

Cancer Prevention. 2017;**18**(1):11-16. DOI: 10.22034/APJCP.2017.18.1.11 [Accessed: October 5, 2020]

[60] Cunha JP. What Will Happen If Endometriosis Is Not Treated? Emedicinehealth. 2019. Available from: https://www.emedicinehealth.com/ask_what_will_happen_if_endometriosis_not_treated/article_em.htm#doctor%E2%80%99s_response [Accessed: October 5, 2020]

[61] Coppa AM. What Happens if Endometriosis is Left Untreated? Available from: https://www.drcoppaobgyn.com/blog/what-happens-if-endometriosis-is-left-untreated

[62] Endometriosis and Ovarian Cancer Risk. Available from: https://ovarian.org.uk/news-and-blog/blog/endometriosis-and-ovarian-cancer-risk/ [Accessed: October 5, 2020]

[63] Reis FM, Coutinho LM, Vannuccini S, Luisi S, Petraglia F. Is stress a cause or a consequence of endometriosis? Reproductive Sciences. 2020;**27**:39-45. DOI: 10.1007/s43032-019-00053-0 [Accessed on October 5, 2020]

[64] Endometriosis vs. Adenomyosis: Similarities and Differences. Available from: https://www.healthline.com/health/womens-health/adenomyosis-vs-endometriosis [Accessed: October 5, 2020]

[65] Endometrial Hyperplasia. Available from: https://my.clevelandclinic.org/health/diseases/16569-atypical-endometrial-hyperplasia [Accessed: October 5, 2020]

Chapter 8

Endometriosis in Mare; What the Mare Can Teach Us When Dealing with Endometriosis in the Woman

David A. Trundell

Abstract

Endometriosis is a serious, often irreversible disease of the mare. Often associated with endometritis, this chapter will review our current understanding of pathophysiology, etiology, diagnosis and possible treatments. Endometriosis is a disease complex typically seen in our older mare population. It is important that we understand that although the same term is used to describe a condition in our human patients, it is, however, not the same medical condition as seen in our equine patients. As this disease profile is irreversible with limited treatment options, it causes significant economic strain in our broodmare population.

Keywords: mare, uterus, endometriosis, endometritis, infertility

1. Introduction

This chapter will examine endometriosis in our equine patients, focusing on etiology, diagnosis/prognosis and treatments for this debilitating condition. Endometriosis in the mare is a multifactorial disease, with severity of endometriosis being positively correlated with age. This condition, although with the same name given to a condition seen in women, is not the same in nature, pathophysiology and/or treatment. A detailed comparison between the condition seen in our equine patients and that of women is given below. Further it is utmost important for the scholars amongst us to be aware of the differences between endometritis and endometriosis; although similar and indeed as will be shown, often linked, they again are different conditions. For clarity, endometritis relates to the inflammation of the endometrium, either of an infectious nature (typically bacteriologic) or noninfectious, such as the presence of spermatozoa in the uterine lumen. Whereas endometriosis in the mare is characterized by chronic endometrial degeneration. This condition has serious consequences from an economic standpoint and often leads to mare being infertile.

2. Etiology and pathophysiology of equine endometriosis

Endometriosis is a debilitating condition leading to significant subfertility and often infertility in the mare, causing significant economic loss in our horse breeding population [1, 2]. The term endometriosis is somewhat misleading in our equine clinics. Endometriosis in the mare is a degenerative, chronic condition demonstrated by fibrosis [3] within the endometrium often as a sequelae to chronic deep

IntechOpen

rooted infection, typically associated with a number of bacterial species. Although this etiology is not universally recognized [4]. This fibrotic condition in the mare is considered irreversible [5–7], and sadly clinicians are limited in their treatment options for this condition. In our human patients, endometriosis is the presence of endometrial glands and stroma-like lesions occurring outside the uterus [8]. These lesions can be peritoneal lesions, superficial implants, cysts on the ovary or deep infiltrating disease in nature [9]. Thus for the academics amongst us, we must understand the difference between our human and non-human patients with regards to the terminology of endometriosis.

Kenney [10] termed endometriosis in our equine patients based on different alterations to the endometrium based on histopathology [11]. A grading system came into effect in the late 1980s [12]; this was later modified by Schoon [12, 13]. Currently endometriosis is defined as active or inactive periglandular and/or stromal endometrial fibrosis including glandular alterations within fibrotic foci [14]. Single glands and/or glandular nests may be affected in equine edometriosis [15, 16]. In our equine patients, endometriosis is further classified as either destructive or non-destructive forms of fibrosis [17]. Endometriosis is a condition that involves the stroma, progressing to involve around the endometrial glands and is characterized by periglandular fibrosis associated with dysfunction of affected glandular epithelial cells [18–20]. Distinguishing between active and inactive, destructive or non-destructive, is based on the morphology of stromal cells involved in fibrotic foci via pathological examination. For the attending veterinarian, regardless of type of endometriosis, the clinical picture would be one of an aged mare, with a history of multiple pregnancies, and pregnancy failure, often with a number of years (recently) of bareness. In tandem these mares are often observed clinically to have endometritis, the hallmark often being hyperechogenic particular fluid within the uterine lumen on transrectal ultrasonography. Destructive endometriosis is characterized by a strong epithelial vimentin expression, excessive extracellular matrix accumulation, cystic gland dilations and mechanical destruction of those glands [21]. Non-destructive endometriosis is characterized by glandular epithelial cells that are intact whereas their degeneration and necrosis are features of destructive endometriosis [22]. Active stromal cells are characterized by an oval shape, pale cytoplasm, and ovoid hypochromatic nuclei whereas inactive stromal cells are spindle shaped with elongated hyperchromatic nuclei [23]. The cyclicity of our mare patients (mares being long day breeders) and associated seasonal endocrine changes appear to have no effect on the disease process.

Mare's age, repeated insult on the endometrium, multiple pregnancies and parturition have been implicated as etiological factors for the development of the degenerative changes within the endometrium seen in endometriosis [24–27]. Nonetheless, not all of these are universally accepted as etiologic factors, as Hoffman [28] found no correlation between endometriosis and number of foaling (i.e. number of pregnancies carried to term), and indeed that of season and estrous cycle associated changes. Older mares with endometriosis have been shown to have a deficient uterine blood flow during pregnancy with poor placenta microvillus development contributing to increased pregnancy loss, or the birth of weak foals [29]; which also reduced fertility in our managed broodmare populations. Further etiologic factors have been described include periglandular localized endometriosis, focal oxygen deficiency (caused by angiosclerosis) and wound healing after mechanical damage leading to physiological turnover of the basal lamina [30]. In a retrospective study by Ebert et al. [31], found that 90 to 92.5% of uterine biopsies showed signs for endometriosis in age categories of 16–20 years and > 20 years of age, respectively.

Following deposition of semen in the uterus, whether by natural service or artificial insemination, a transient inflammatory process is initiated within the uterus. This is a normal physiologic event in the mare. This process removes excessive spermatozoa and bacteria that may be induced in the uterus are removed. This process peaks some 12 hours after deposition of semen within the uterus, and is usually completed within 48 hours after insult [32]. It has been suggested that this mechanism of uterine clearance is a critical factor in the uterine defense against infection [33].

Mares susceptible to endometritis have difficulty in clearing inflammatory debris either due to anatomical and/or degenerative defects that interfere with uterine drainage. These defects include a pendulous uterus, impaired myometrium contractility, lymphatic or cervical drainage, atrophy of endometrial folds and disturbed mucociliary clearance. It has been postulated that this decreased physical clearance may increase endometrial periglandular fibrosis [34] and result in decreased pregnancy rates in the mare. There is consensus amongst authorities that there is an initial insult to the endometrium, whether bacteriologic in nature or not, that triggers the start of a complex pathophysiologic process, ending in endometriosis [35–39]. Nonetheless, there are some underlying risk factors to the development of endometriosis. In the initial stages of endometriosis, stromal cells synthesize collagen fibers and differentiate into myofibroblasts, which in turn are responsible for extracellular matrix deposition, eventually ending in endometrial periglandular fibrosis [40]. Periglandular-accentuated mononuclear cell infiltrates (PAMC) have also been suggested as a possible triggering event to endometriosis development [41].

Once established, the endometrium is characterized by abundant fibrosis, ulcer-like holes present on the surface of the epithelium; the cells lack cilia, have few organelles and increased degenerative cell structures [42]. In spite of extensive tissue damage seen in endometriosis, cyclic vascular and non-vascular tissue growth occurs in a coordinated manner as in non-affected mares [43]. Different types of endometriosis are a reflection of different stages of fibrotic process [44]. These areas (endometriosis-affected) of the endometrium exhibit specific differentiation dynamics and become independent from normal uterine control mechanism [45]. Nonetheless, the cardinal feature of endometriosis according to Walter [46] is the deposition of extracellular matrix by myofibroblasts located around the endometrial glands. The epithelial differentiation of the fibrotic uterine glands can be divided into a cycle synchronous, asynchronous and intermediate forms [47]. Initially an epithelial hypertrophy with subsequent epithelial degeneration and glandular dilatation with congestion of secretions is observed, as well as epithelial cell atrophy; there are marked differences in several epithelial enzymatic secretion pathways in the fibrotic foci compared to unaffected glands [48]. Hoffman [49] found that there is a temporary activation of fibrotic stromal cells which were observed after experimentally induced bacterial endometritis likely mediated via profibrotic growth factors and cytokines released by inflammatory cells.

The precise mechanism of endometriosis in the mare is not yet fully understood despite many decades of research. It appears that there is an initial insult, whether non-infectious such as deposition of semen within the uterus or bacterial in origin, results in neutrophil (PMN) migration into the uterine lumen [50]. PMN are the first line of defense (part of the innate immune defense system) against invading microorganisms [51].

It should be noted that endometriosis does not appear to impair PMN functionality [52]. In susceptible mares (in relation to endometritis), those that have a IIB and III endometrial score of biopsy (**Table 1**) have a significant influx of PMN two to twenty-four hours post insult to the endometrium. This PMN hyperactivation and its role in causing severe inflammation and their role in the progression of endometriosis is not fully unknown [54]. PMN appear to cast off the DNA in response to infectious stimuli, forming neutrophil extracellular traps (NETs) [55]. These consist of DNA associated molecule complexes which transport nucleic and cytoplasmic

Category	Histological findings	Estimated foaling rates (to produce a live foal)
I	No significant alterations	>80–90%
IIa	Mild endometritis OR Mild endometriosis OR Mild lymphatic lacunae OR Partial endometrial atrophy during late breeding season	50–80%
IIb	Moderate endometritis OR Moderate endometriosis OR Moderate lymphatic lacunae OR Bareness >2 years OR A combination of two categories from IIa findings	10–50%
III	Marked endometritis OR Marked endometriosis OR Marked lymphatic lacunae OR Deep endometrial atrophy during the breeding season OR Combined presence of three or more IIa findings or 2 or more IIb/III findings	<10%

Table 1.
Categorization of endometrial score proposed by Kenny and Doig [53] and modified by Schoon et al. [12].

proteins, which appear to have immunomodulating properties [56]. PMN play a positive role in infection control, however, they can also have a deleterious effect by their content releasing molecules, which can alter the endometrium potentially contributing to the formation of fibrosis on the endometrium architecture [57].

In inflamed tissues, an intricate network of pro-fibrotic cytokines interacts with extracellular matrix, fibroblasts and other cells to regulate collagen deposition and tissue fibrosis [58]. It is known that in the mare with endometriosis, those that are susceptible to endometritis, there is a release of pro-inflammatory cytokines, including interleukins (IL-1B) and TNFα - both of which have high mRNA expression [59]. However, early in the post insemination period a lower mRNA expression of IL-6 and IL-10 were detected in susceptible PMIE (post mating induced endometritis) mares [60]. Included in that study were mares diagnosed with endometriosis. In a further study, it was shown that *E. coli* induced endometritis showed a sustained expression of pro-inflammatory cytokines (IL-1β and IL-8) within the endometrium [61]. Thus it can be suggested that these disturbed expressions of endometrial inflammatory cytokines may play a role in the pathogenesis of endometriosis [62]. Researchers have found that expression levels of IL1RA (an interleukin receptor antagonist) were lower in endometriosis affected endometria compared with non-affected endometria, suggesting a protective role with the endometrium [63].

The first signs of endometriosis on histopathomorphology are atypical morphology and functional differentiation of periglandular stromal cells [64]. The first stage of fibrosis is characterized by large polygonal periglandular stromal cells (type 1) that synthesize collagen fibers [65]. In advanced fibrosis, metabolic active or inactive stromal cells (type II) without signs of collagen synthesis, as well as myofibroblasts, predominate [66]. In the latter, the contractability appears to be affected and may lead to a constriction of uterine glands resulting in glandular dilation [67]. Additionally myofibroblasts may be able to affect the composition and amount of extracellular matrix by secreting different mediators [68]. Typically the endometrium undergoes cyclic changes with typical histomorphological, ezymethistochemical and immunohistocehmical glandular patterns in response to steroid levels [69]. The changes observed in endometriosis on histopathology are independent of the stage of the estrous cycle.

A number of researchers have examined the alteration in secretion pattern of a number of uterine enzymes, namely uteroglobin, uterocalin, calbindin, uteroferrin, and their potential role in the pathogenesis of endometriosis [70–76]. Uteroclain is the most prominent progesterone dependent uterine derived protein, which is abundantly expressed during pregnancy [77]. Uteroglobin, also progesterone dependent and of uterine origin, is thought to mask the trophoblasts from the mare's immune system, allowing pregnancy to establish [78]. Calbindin$_{D9K}$ is a small cytosolic protein expressed by the endometrium, and has a role in the transport of calcium from glandular epithelia and from the blood supply to the uterine lumen [79]. Uteroferrin again is a endometrial derived progesterone dependent protein that is involved with iron transport during pregnancy [80]. Hoffman [81] showed a synchronous expression pattern: uterocallin and uteroglobin expression were decreased, whereas uteroferrin expression was increased in affected glandular epithelia. Lehman [82] found that affected endometria showed decreased fibrotic stromal cell expression of both estrogen and progesterone receptors compared to unaffected endometria. Normal cyclic dependent expression of these proteins were not observed in affected endometrial tissue, however what is observed is within fibrotic foci, there is a cycle asynchronous patchy protein secretion [83]. Hoffman [84] observed a decrease in uterocallin expression in mares suffering from both destructive and non-destructive fibrosis of their endometrium. Hoffman [85] found that there was decreased expression of Calbindin$_{D9K}$ in fibrotic glands of the endometrium; however, this was not observed by Lehman [86] and therefore is an unreliable marker for endometriosis in the mare. Lehman [87] concluded that uterogoblin and uterocallin should be utilized when trying to refine biopsy classification of endometrium biopsy for our mare population.

Two enzymes that are secreted in abundance in the process of fibrosis in the endometrium, that are capable of degrading collagen IV and laminin, are Tissue Transglutaminase (TG2) and Matrix Metalloproteinase (MMP2) [88]. These enzymes have also been implicated in causing dilation of uterine glands [89]. However, although these enzymes have been implicated in fibrosis, there is contradictory evidence to suggest that there is no correlation between the secretion of these enzymes and the development of endometriosis in the mare [90]. MMP-9 has been shown to degrade collagen IV, the main component of basement membranes [91]. In humans MMP-9 has been reported to be expressed in inflammatory cells as well as glandular and periglandular stromal cells in the endometrium [92].

In a two year experiment where mares were subjected to induced and repeated endometritis researchers found that these endometritis events had no significant exacerbation of the endometriosis observed [93]. Hoffman [94] found in the equine endometrium distinctly reduced ER (estrogen receptors) and PR (progesterone receptors) expression; in fibrotic stromal cells as compared to the unaltered stroma and these markers according to Hoffman [95] are the hallmarks of equine endometriosis. Studies in human patients with endometriosis have found similar results. On the microscopic level it has been reported that the hallmark of endometriosis in the mare is the appearance of concentric arrangement of stromal cells and/or collagen fibers around affected glands [96]. The degree of periglandular fibrosis is determined by the number of periglandular layers of stromal cells and the number of fibrotic nests of glands [97].

Hoffman [98] observed that there is accumulation of fibronectin and proteoglycans particularly in active destructive fibrotic foci and is probably due to an increased number of secretively active myofibroblasts. Hoffman [99] suggests a pathogenesis of endometriosis which the authors describe as conceivable; there is an initial epithelial alteration and activation with a partial thickening of the affected parts of the basal lamina. Only an intact basal lamina is able to suppress the epithelial cell activation and the synthesis of profibrotic growth factors [100]. The early stages of fibrosis are characterized by slight basal lamina alterations with a focal accumulation of stromal cells which synthesize collagen fibers [101].

It has been described in equine endometriosis that there is stromal cell proliferation and their differentiation into myofibroblasts as well as their increased synthesis of extracellular matrix (ECM) occurs in response to a milieu of synergistically and autoinductively acting mediators which might result in a periglandular fibrosis [102].

With different grades of endometriosis, increasing amounts of collagen IV are deposited around the endometrial glands and fibrotic nests [103]. Aresu [104] hypothesized that MMP-9 production would increase with endometriosis; however their results showed no significant increase in this protein level with endometriosis affected mares and controls. They concluded that immunohistochemistry is not useful in clinical practice to evaluate fertility. Hoffman [105] has concluded that it does seem as though endometritis is the initiator to activate the process of endometriosis.

There is clear evidence between age and the degree of endometriosis observed in our equine patients; however the degree of inflammation and grade of endometriosis is poorly correlated [106]. Fibrosis continues to progress even after the inflammatory process has stopped [107]. Therefore this process becomes independent of the initial inflammatory event of which it arose from.

3. Role of prostaglandins in the pathogenesis of equine endometriosis

It has been demonstrated that fibrosis of the lungs is often the result of low grade, chronic inflammation, and this may be true in the development of endometriosis [108]. In addition to the cytokines described above, the role of eicosanoids including prostaglandin E_2 and $F_{2\alpha}$ could provide an alternative pathway to fibrogenesis [109].

The short half-life of prostaglandins would suggest that they act locally via specific receptors [110]. When PGE_2 binds to its E prostanoid receptor it triggers numerous antifibrotic events within fibroblasts, epithelial cells and leukocytes. However when it binds to $PGF_{2\alpha}$ receptors (to which it has lower affinity) it induces fibrosis with lung tissue. In the woman, there is emerging evidence of the role of PG and the development of fibrosis, with PG receptors providing a signaling pathway for their enzymes to cause vasoconstriction, increase myometrial contractions and pain [111]. It has been shown in the mare's endometrium, those suffering with endometriosis, there is altered synthesis of PG and mRNA transcription of prostaglandin synthases [112]. In i*n vitro* studies, it has been shown that decreased PGE_2 production coupled with an increase in mRNA type 1 collagen level due to sustained, low grade chronic infectious stimulus may establish a pathway to endometrial fibrosis [113].

NETs have been shown to decrease prostaglandin E_2 that exerts an antifibrotic response after binding to the E prostanoid receptor [114]. It has been suggested that mares with underlying endometriosis predisposes the uterus to endometritis, rather than the other way around. This is based on observations that *in vitro* induced bacterial endometritis with subsequent treatments was not associated with the progression of endometriosis over a 2 year observation period in 90% of the mares. Whether endometritis is the initiator to endometriosis or vice versa, a mutual influence of endometritis and endometriosis has been postulated by a number of authors [115].

Hoffman [116] found that advanced dedifferentiation of the stromal cells within the fibrotic foci led to inadequate hormone receptor expression that are not able to react to cyclic endocrine changes, becoming independent of hormonal control mechanisms in the uterus.

The establishment of equine endometriosis is a dynamic and complicated process, involving PMN, their role in NETs production and the release of their contents, pro-fibrotic cytokines, interleukins and PG production.

4. Diagnosis

Uterine biopsy is a standard test to evaluate the endometrium, to grade it and most importantly to give the clinician a prognosis of likelihood of the mare to carry a pregnancy to term. This is an indispensable test for evaluating fertility in our mares. Endometrial Biopsy are used to evaluate endometrial health, presence and degree of uterine disease and as a prognostic indicator to future fertility of our equine patients. Evaluation of the degree of endometrial fibrosis is essential as, in contrast to the inflammatory changes, fibrosis is of a permanent nature, and, if it is intense, it becomes the main factor that reduces the reproductive performance of the mare [117].

A detailed description and step by step guide to obtaining a biopsy from a mare's uterus is provided in the book Equine Reproductive Procedures [118], however a brief overview is provided here. It is recommended that a transrectal ultrasound is performed prior to obtaining a biopsy, especially in unknown mares, to rule out concurrent pregnancy. It is also recommended to obtain the sample in either diestrus or early estrus (confirmed by transrectal ultrasonography) and this information should be supplied to the pathologists, to allow for normal alterations of the endometrium due to stage of the estrous cycle to be considered.

The perineum should be thoroughly washed with a non-residual soap and rinsed clean with clean water, and dried with disposable tissue. A sterile obstetrical sleeve with sterile lubricant is worn by the veterinarian, and with the biopsy instrument in a closed position is advanced through the vagina, and carefully through the cervix, with the examiners hand acting as both a guide and protector to the delicate tissues of the reproductive tract. The veterinarian removes his arm from the vagina and inserts it rectally; this is to guide the instrument to the correct location for sampling typically at the base of either of the uterine horns. The biopsy instrument is carefully opened, and with a ventral pressure from the rectum, the endometrial tissue is forced into the cutting basket of the instrument. The examiner then closes the instrument and retracts it from the vagina. The small sample of uterine tissue is then placed into a fixative solution such as 10% formalin or Bouin's solution. The container should be labeled appropriately and sent to the pathologists for interpretation. A single biopsy from this area has been shown to be representative of the entire endometrium [118]. A slight hemorrhagic discharge from the vulva may be seen up to 24 hours post biopsy, and owners should be informed of such.

5. Treatment

There is no satisfactory treatment for equine endometriosis and this is frustrating for all clinicians working within equine theriogenology. The changes to the endometrium are considered by most authorities to be irreversible. However, there is some anecdotal evidence for treatments that revolve around mechanical curettage or use of chemical agents such as kerosene, DMSO and isotonic salts which may be beneficial [119]. Analysis of physical curettage applied to mares will typically cause hyperemia within the endometrium and lead to establishment of endometritis, which can be treated utilizing appropriate antibiotic therapy based on culture and sensitivity. After treatment mares treated with kerosene intrauterine showed an improved biopsy score; 44% increase, 51% no change, and 5% showed a deterioration of grade [120]. Kerosene is widely used in broodmare practice to potentially revert uterine fibrosis, via endometrial necrosis.

A detailed description and step by step guide to lavaging a mare's uterus is provided in the book Equine Reproductive Procedures [121], however a brief overview is provided here. The mare is retained in adequate stocks, and can be sedated if required. Her tail should be wrapped and held to the side to allow visualization and access to the vulva, without the possibility of contamination from her tail. The vulva and surrounding perineum is washed with a non-residue soap and rinsed. It is then dried with disposal paper. The clinician should put on a sterile, disposal glove and a small amount of sterile lubricant applied to the back of the gloved hand. The assistant should open the sterile y-tubing, avoiding contamination and allow the veterinarian to put the tubing end into his/her hand. The other end of the tubing should be connected to a fluid bag containing approximately 500 mL kerosene. The clinician should open the clasp to allow some kerosene to run through the tubing before it is entered into the uterus to prevent instilling air into the uterus. The clinician should alert the horse of their presence by gently patting the mare of her side with his/her ungloved hand. The sterile glove containing the lubricant should be slowly introduced through the vulva, avoiding any contamination. Clasp the hand around the end of the tubing as you advance through the cervix; this will protect the delicate mucosa from any potential damage. Once the cervix has been located, slowly advance the tubing into the uterus. Utilizing the hand that is inside the mare gently clasp the cervix closed around the tubing and begin instilling the kerosene. Approximately 500 mL should be infused into the uterus. Once delivered, slowly remove your arm from the mare's reproductive tract. Leave the kerosene in the mare for approximately 24 hours.

The following day the mare is returned to the stocks, and her perineum is cleaned as above. The mare is then subjected to a uterine lavage, utilizing Lactated Ringer's solution (LRS). Initially the fluid that is returned from the uterus is cloudy often with particular matter - these are sloughed off parts of the endometrium. Continue to lavage the uterus until the returned fluid runs clear. This may be several liters. Often it is recommended to repeat the uterine lavage the next day. The clinician may utilize the aid of ecbolic agents such as oxytocin given I.V. or I.M. (one unit) to aid in the evacuation of uterine contents.

6. Concluding remarks

Endometriosis is often linked to endometritis in our mare patients. This frustrating disease complex is irreversible and debilitating for the mare and owner alike. This condition once diagnosed leaves the clinician with little options when it comes to treatment choices. Although strides have been made in utilizing enzymatic and protein detection in biopsy sampling for grading of the uterus, this, unfortunately offers the clinician little in terms of possible treatments. Any mare suspected to be suffering from endometriosis should have a uterine biopsy performed. This allows for classification, grading and prognosis, which will help the practitioner to have educated discussions with the mare's owner. If the clinician at hand is working on sport horses, such as show jumpers or quarter horses, options include embryo transfer or intracytoplasmic sperm injection (ICSI). However, should the clinician be working on thoroughbreds for racing, all worldwide jurisdictions ban such measures, and the mare must carry and deliver her own offspring. In these situations, faced with a mare with endometriosis, leaves the veterinarian with little option but to try chemical lavages as described above, such as kerosene uterine lavage. However, prior to this a biopsy should be obtained to confirm endometriosis, and to allow the clinician to clearly and precisely explain to the owner of the mare, the mare's likelihood of carrying a foal to term.

Author details

David A. Trundell
DT Veterinary Services, Skelmuir, United Kingdom

*Address all correspondence to: dt.vet2020@gmail.com

References

[1] Hoffman C, Ellenberger C, Mattos RC et al.: The equine endometriosis: new insights into the pathogenesis. Animal Reproductive Science. 2009;3(2-4): 261-278. DOI:10.1016/j.anireprosci.2008.03.019.

[2] Aresu L, Benali S, Giannuzzi D, et al.: The role of inflammation and matrix metalloproteinases in equine reproduction. Journal of Veterinary Science. 2005;13(2):171-177 DOI:10.4142/jvs.2012.13.2.171.

[3] Szostek-Miduchowska AZ, Baclawska A, Okuda K, Skarzynski DJ. Effect of proinflammatory cytokines on endometrial collagen and metallopeptidase expression during the course of equine endometriosis. J. Cytokine. 2019;123:154767 DOI: https://doi.org/10.1016/j.cyto.2019.154767.

[4] Rebordao MR, Galvo A, Szotek A, et al. Physiopathologic mechanisms involved in mare endometriosis. Reprod Dom Anim. 2014;49(4):82-87 DOI: :https://doi.org/10.1111/rda.12397

[5] Kenney RM. The aetiology, diagnosis and classification of chronic degenerative endometritis. In Hughes JP (ed.), Workshop on equine endometritis. 1992;125:186

[6] Hoffman C, Ellenberger C, Mattos RC et al.: The equine endometriosis: new insights into the pathogenesis. Animal Reproductive Science. 2009;3(2-4): 261-278 DOI: 10.1016/j.anireprosci.2008.03.019

[7] Aresu L, Benali S, Giannuzzi D, et al.: The role of inflammation and matrix metalloproteinases in equine reproduction. Journal of Veterinary Science. 2005;13(2):171-177. DOI: 10.4142/jvs.2012.13.2.171

[8] Giudice LC, Kao LC. Endometriosis. Lancet. 2004;364(9447):1789-1799.

[9] Nisolle M, Donnez J. Peritoneal endometriosis, ovarian endometriosis, and adenomyotic nodules of the rectovaginal septum are three different entities. Fert Steril. 1997;68(4):585-596. DOI: 10.1016/s0015-0282(97)00191-x.

[10] Kenney RM. The aetiology, diagnosis and classification of chronic degenerative endometritis. In Hughes JP (ed.), Workshop on equine endometritis. 1992;125:186.

[11] Kenney RM. Cyclic and pathological changes of the mare endometrium as detected by biopsy, with a note on early embryonic death. J AM Vet Med Assoc. 1978;172:241-262. PMID: 621166.

[12] Schoon, H.-A.; Schoon, D.; Klug, E. Uterusbiopsien als Hilfsmittel für Diagnose und Prognose von Fertilitätsstörungen der Stute. Pferdeheilkunde 1992, 8, 355-362.

[13] Schoon, H.-A.; Schoon, D.; Klug, E. Die Endometriumbiopsie bei der Stute im klinisch-gynäkologischen Kontext. Pferdeheilkunde 1997, 13, 453-464.

[14] Hanada M, Michiko Y, Oikawa MA. Histopathological characteristics of endometriosis in thoroughbred mares in Japan: results from 50 necropsy cases. Journal of equine science. 2014.25(2): 45-52. doi:10.1294/jes.25.45. DOI:10.1294/jes.25.45.

[15] Schöniger S, Schoon HA. The Healthy and Diseased Equine Endometrium: A Review of Morphological Features and Molecular Analyses. Animals (Basel). 2020;10(4):625. doi: 10.3390/ani10040625.

[16] Kenney RM. Cyclic and pathological changes of the mare endometrium as detected by biopsy, with a note on early embryonic death. J AM Vet Med Assoc. 1978;172:241-262. PMID: 621166.

[17] Lehmann J, Ellenberger C, Hoffman C et al. Morpho-functional studies regarding the fertility prognosis of mares suffering from equine endometriosis. Theriogenology. 2011;76:1326-1336

[18] Doig PA, McKnight JD, Miller RB. The use of endometrial biopsy in the infertile mare. Can Vet J. 1981;22:72-76. PMID: 7026016

[19] Hoffman C, Ellenberger C, Mattos RC et al.: The equine endometriosis: new insights into the pathogenesis. Animal Reproductive Science. 2009;3(2-4): 261-278 DOI:10.1016/j.anireprosci. 2008.03.019.

[20] Walter I, Handler J, Reifinger M, Aurich C. Association of endometriosis in horses with differentiation of periglandular myofibroblasts and changes of extracellular matrix protein. Reproduction. 2001;121:581-586. PMID: 11277878.

[21] Hoffman C, Ellenberger C, Mattos RC et al.: The equine endometriosis: new insights into the pathogenesis. Animal Reproductive Science. 2009;3(2-4): 261-278. DOI:10.1016/j.anireprosci. 2008.03.019.

[22] Schöniger S, Schoon HA. The Healthy and Diseased Equine Endometrium: A Review of Morphological Features and Molecular Analyses. Animals (Basel). 2020;10(4):625. doi: 10.3390/ ani10040625.

[23] ovoid hypochromatic nuclei whereas inactive stromal cells are spindle shaped with elongated hyperchromatic nuclei

[24] Doig PA, McKnight JD, Miller RB. The use of endometrial biopsy in the infertile mare. Can Vet J. 1981;22:72-76.

[25] Hoffmann C Bazer FW, Klug J, Aupperle H, Ellenberger C, Schoon HA. Immunohistochemical and histochemical identification of proteins and carbohydrates in the equine endometrium expression patterns for mares suffering from endometriosis. Theriogenology. 2009;71:264-274.

[26] LeBlanc MM, Causey RC. Clinical and subclinical endometritis in the mare: both threats to fertility. Reprod Dom Anim. 2009;44(3):10-22.

[27] Ricketts SW, Alonso S. The effect of age and parity on the development of equine chronic endometrial disease. Equine Vet J. 1991;23:189-192.

[28] Hoffman C, Ellenberger C, Mattos RC et al.: The equine endometriosis: new insights into the pathogenesis. Animal Reproductive Science. 2009;3(2-4): 261-278 DOI:10.1016/j.anireprosci. 2008.03.019.

[29] Ousey JC, Kolling M, Newton R, Wright M, Allen, WR Uterine haemodynamics in young and aged pregnant mares measured using Doppler ultrasonography. Equine Veterinary Journal.2012;44:15-21. https://doi. org/10.1111/j.2042-3306.2011.00446.x

[30] Hoffman C, Ellenberger C, Mattos RC et al.: The equine endometriosis: new insights into the pathogenesis. Animal Reproductive Science. 2009;3(2-4):261-278.

[31] Ebert A., Schoon D., Schoon H.-A. Age-related endometrial alterations in mares—biopsy findings of the last 20 years. In: Rackwitz R., Pees M., Aschenbach J.R., Gäbel G., editors. Leipziger Blaue Hefte, 7th Leipzig Veterinary Congress, 8th International Conference on Equine Reproductive Medicine. Volume 2. Lehmanns Media GmbH; Berlin, Germany: 2014. pp. 230-232.

[32] Katila T. Uterine defence mechanisms in the mare. Animal Reproduction Science. 1996;42:197-204. doi: 10.1016/0378-4320(96)01507-2

[33] LeBlanc MM, Causey RC. Clinical and subclinical endometritis in the mare: both threats to fertility. Reprod Dom Anim. 2009;44(3):10-22.

[34] Schöniger S, Schoon HA. The Healthy and Diseased Equine Endometrium: A Review of Morphological Features and Molecular Analyses. Animals (Basel). 2020 Apr 5;10(4):625. doi: 10.3390/ani10040625. PMID: 32260515; PMCID: PMC7222714.

[35] Szóstek AZ, Lukasik K, Galvão AM, Ferreira-Dias GM, Skarzynski DJ. Impairment of the interleukin system in equine endometrium during the course of endometriosis. Biol Reprod. 2013;89(4):79. doi: 10.1095/biolreprod.113.109447.

[36] Amaral A, Fernandes C, Lukasik K, Szóstek-Mioduchowska A, Baclawska A, Rebordão MR, Aguiar-Silva J, Pinto-Bravo P, Skarzynski DJ, Ferreira-Dias G. Elastase inhibition affects collagen transcription and prostaglandin secretion in mare endometrium during the estrous cycle. Reprod Domest Anim. 2018;53(2):66-69. doi: 10.1111/rda.13258.

[37] Rebordão MR, Amaral A, Lukasik K, Szóstek-Mioduchowska A, Pinto-Bravo P, Galvão A, Skarzynski DJ, Ferreira-Dias G. Constituents of neutrophil extracellular traps induce in vitro collagen formation in mare endometrium. Theriogenology. 2018;113:8-18. doi: 10.1016/j.theriogenology.2018.02.001.

[38] Szóstek-Mioduchowska AZ, Lukasik K, Skarzynski DJ, Okuda K. Effect of transforming growth factor -β1 on α-smooth muscle actin and collagen expression in equine endometrial fibroblasts, Theriogenology. 2019;124:9-17, https://doi.org/10.1016/j.theriogenology.2018.10.005.

[39] Rebordão MR, Amaral A, Lukasik K, Szóstek-Mioduchowska A, Pinto-Bravo P, Galvão A, Skarzynski DJ, Ferreira-Dias G. Impairment of the antifibrotic prostaglandin E2 pathway may influence neutrophil extracellular traps-induced fibrosis in the mare endometrium. Domest Anim Endocrinol. 2019;67:1-10. doi: 10.1016/j.domaniend.2018.10.004.

[40] Raila G. Zur Pathogenese der Endometrose der Stute - Morphologisch-funktionelle Untersuchungen. Diss. Med. Vet. Leipzig. 2000.

[41] Klose, K.; Schoon, H.-A. Periglandular inflammatory cells in the endometrium of the mare—A physiological defence mechanisms which impacts on the development of endometriosis. Pferdeheilkunde 2016, 32, 15-23

[42] Rebordão, M, Galvão, A, Szóstek, A, Amaral, A, Mateus, L, Skarzynski, D, Ferreira-Dias, G. Physiopathologic Mechanisms Involved in Mare Endometriosis. Reprod Dom Anim, 49: 82-87. https://doi.org/10.1111/rda.12397

[43] Rebordão, M, Galvão, A, Szóstek, A, Amaral, A, Mateus, L, Skarzynski, D, Ferreira-Dias, G. Physiopathologic Mechanisms Involved in Mare Endometriosis. Reprod Dom Anim, 49: 82-87. https://doi.org/10.1111/rda.12397

[44] Hoffmann C, Ellenberger C, Mattos RC, Aupperle H, Dhein S, Stief B, Schoon HA. The equine endometriosis: new insights into the pathogenesis. Anim Reprod Sci. 2009;111: 261– 278. DOI:10.1016/j.anireprosci.2008.03.019.

[45] Lehmann J, Ellenberger C, Hoffmann C, Bazer FW, Klug J, Allen WR, Sieme H, Schoon HA. Morpho-functional studies regarding the fertility prognosis of mares suffering from equine endometriosis. Theriogenology. 2011;76(7):1326-1336. doi: 10.1016/j.theriogenology.2011.06.001.

[46] Walter I, Handler J, Miller I, Aurich C. Matrix metalloproteinase 2 (MMP-2) and tissue transglutaminase (TG 2) are expressed in periglandular fibrosis in horse mares with endometriosis. Histol Histopathol. 2005;20(4):1105-13. doi: 10.14670/HH-20.1105.

[47] Schöniger S, Schoon HA. The Healthy and Diseased Equine Endometrium: A Review of Morphological Features and Molecular Analyses. Animals (Basel). 2020;10(4):625. DOI:10.3390/ani10040625

[48] Lehmann J, Ellenberger C, Hoffmann C, Bazer FW, Klug J, Allen WR, Sieme H, Schoon HA. Morpho-functional studies regarding the fertility prognosis of mares suffering from equine endometriosis. Theriogenology. 2011;76(7):1326-1336. doi: 10.1016/j.theriogenology.2011.06.001.

[49] Hoffmann C, Ellenberger C, Mattos RC, Aupperle H, Dhein S, Stief B, Schoon HA. The equine endometriosis: new insights into the pathogenesis. Anim Reprod Sci. 2009;111: 261– 278

[50] Troedsson MH, Liu IK, Thurmond M. Function of uterine and blood-derived polymorphonuclear neutrophils in mares susceptible and resistant to chronic uterine infection: phagocytosis and chemotaxis. Biol Reprod. 1993;49(3):507-514. doi: 10.1095/biolreprod49.3.507.

[51] LeBlanc, M. (2010), Advances in the Diagnosis and Treatment of Chronic Infectious and Post–Mating-Induced Endometritis in the Mare. Reproduction in Domestic Animals.2010;45: 21-27. https://doi.org/10.1111/j.1439-0531.2010.01634.x

[52] Rebordão, M, Galvão, A, Szóstek, A, Amaral, A, Mateus, L, Skarzynski, D, Ferreira-Dias, G. Physiopathologic Mechanisms Involved in Mare endometriosis. Reprod Dom Anim, 49: 82-87. https://doi.org/10.1111/rda.12397

[53] Kenny RM, Doig PA. Equine endometrial biopsy, in DA Morrow (Hrsg): current therapy in theriogenology 2 Philadelphia, WB Saunder, comp. 1986.

[54] Rebordão, M, Galvão, A, Szóstek, A, Amaral, A, Mateus, L, Skarzynski, D, Ferreira-Dias, G. Physiopathologic Mechanisms Involved in Mare endometriosis. Reprod Dom Anim, 49: 82-87. https://doi.org/10.1111/rda.12397

[55] Rebordão, M, Galvão, A, Szóstek, A, Amaral, A, Mateus, L, Skarzynski, D, Ferreira-Dias, G. Physiopathologic Mechanisms Involved in Mare endometriosis. Reprod Dom Anim, 49: 82-87. https://doi.org/10.1111/rda.12397

[56] Rebordão, M, Galvão, A, Szóstek, A, Amaral, A, Mateus, L, Skarzynski, D, Ferreira-Dias, G. Physiopathologic Mechanisms Involved in Mare endometriosis. Reprod Dom Anim, 49: 82-87. https://doi.org/10.1111/rda.12397

[57] Lögters T, Margraf S, Altrichter J, Cinatl J, Mitzner S, Windolf J, Scholz M. The clinical value of neutrophil extracellular traps. Med Microbiol Immunol. 2009;198(4):211-219. doi: 10.1007/s00430-009-0121-x.

[58] Atamas SP. Complex cytokine regulation of tissue fibrosis. Life Sci. 2002 Dec 27;72(6):631-643. doi: 10.1016/s0024-3205(02)02299-3.

[59] Fumuso E, Giguère S, Wade J, Rogan D, Videla-Dorna I, Bowden RA. Endometrial IL-1beta, IL-6 and TNF-alpha, mRNA expression in mares resistant or susceptible to post-breeding endometritis. Effects of estrous cycle, artificial insemination and immunomodulation. Vet Immunol Immunopathol. 2003;96(1-2):31-41. DOI: 10.1016/s0165-2427(03)00137-5.

[60] Woodward EM, Christoffersen M, Campos J, Betancourt A, Horohov D, Scoggin KE, Squires EL, Troedsson MH. Endometrial inflammatory markers of the early immune response in mares susceptible or resistant to persistent breeding-induced endometritis. Reproduction. 2013 Mar 1;145(3):289-296. DOI: 10.1530/rep-12-0452.

[61] Christoffersen, M., Woodward, E., Bojesen, A.M. et al. Inflammatory responses to induced infectious endometritis in mares resistant or susceptible to persistent endometritis. BMC Vet Res. 2012;8:41. https://doi.org/10.1186/1746-6148-8-41

[62] Christoffersen, M., Woodward, E., Bojesen, A.M. et al. Inflammatory responses to induced infectious endometritis in mares resistant or susceptible to persistent endometritis. BMC Vet Res. 2012;8:41. https://doi.org/10.1186/1746-6148-8-41

[63] Christoffersen, M., Woodward, E., Bojesen, A.M. et al. Inflammatory responses to induced infectious endometritis in mares resistant or susceptible to persistent endometritis. BMC Vet Res. 2012;8:41. https://doi.org/10.1186/1746-6148-8-41

[64] Hoffmann C, Ellenberger C, Mattos RC, Aupperle H, Dhein S, Stief B, Schoon HA. The equine endometriosis: new insights into the pathogenesis. Anim Reprod Sci. 2009;111: 261– 278. DOI:10.1016/j.anireprosci.2008.03.019.

[65] Hoffmann C, Ellenberger C, Mattos RC, Aupperle H, Dhein S, Stief B, Schoon HA. The equine endometriosis: new insights into the pathogenesis. Anim Reprod Sci. 2009;111: 261– 278

[66] Raila G. Zur Pathogenese der Endometrose der Stute - Morphologisch-funktionelle Untersuchungen. Diss. Med. Vet. Leipzig. 2000.

[67] Hoffmann C, Ellenberger C, Mattos RC, Aupperle H, Dhein S, Stief B, Schoon HA. The equine endometriosis: new insights into the pathogenesis. Anim Reprod Sci. 2009;111: 261– 278. DOI:10.1016/j.anireprosci.2008.03.019.DOI:10.1016/j.anireprosci.2008.03.019.

[68] Evans TJ, Miller MA, Ganjam VK, Niswender KD, Ellersieck MR, Krause WJ, Youngquist RS. Morphometric analysis of endometrial periglandular fibrosis in mares. Am J Vet Res. 1998 Oct;59(10):1209-1214. PMID: 9781449.

[69] Brunckhorst, D. & Schoon, H.-A & Bader, Hassaan & Sieme, H.. (1991). Morphologische, enzym- und immunhistochemische Charakteristika des endometrialen Zyklus bei der Stute. Fertilität. 7. 44-51.

[70] Hoffman C. Morphologisch-funktionelle Untersuchungen zur Pathogenese der equinen Endometrose unter besonderer Berücksichtigung endometrialer Proteine und Kohlenhydrate[dissertation vet. med.]. 2006. Leipzig.

[71] Hoffmann C, Bazer F, Klug J, Aupperle H, Ellenberger C, Schoon HA. Schoon. Immunohistochemical and histochemical identification of proteins and carbohydrates in the equine endometrium: reaction patterns in the cycling mare. DOI: Pferdeheilkunde. 2009.25:212-219.10.1016/j.theriogenology.2008.07.008.

[72] Ellenberger C, Wilsher S, Allen WR, Hoffmann C, Kölling M, Bazer FW, Klug J, Schoon D, Schoon HA. Immunolocalisation of the uterine secretory proteins uterocalin, uteroferrin and uteroglobin in the mare's uterus and placenta throughout pregnancy. Theriogenology. 2008 Sep

15;70(5):746-757. doi: 10.1016/j. theriogenology.2008.04.050.

[73] Stewart, Fabian & Kennedy, M & Suire, Sabine. (2000). A novel uterine lipocalin supporting pregnancy in equids. Cellular and molecular life sciences: CMLS. 57. 1373-8. DOI:10.1007/PL00000622.

[74] Hoffmann C, Bazer F, Klug J, Aupperle H, Ellenberger C, Schoon HA. Schoon. Immunohistochemical and histochemical identification of proteins and carbohydrates in the equine endometrium: reaction patterns in the cycling mare. Pferdeheilkunde.2009.25:212-219. DOI:10.1016/j.theriogenology. 2008.07.008.

[75] Lehmann J, Ellenberger C, Hoffmann C, Bazer FW, Klug J, Allen WR, Sieme H, Schoon HA. Morpho-functional studies regarding the fertility prognosis of mares suffering from equine endometriosis. Theriogenology. 2011;76(7):1326-1336. doi:10.1016/j.theriogenology.2011.06.001.

[76] Roberts RM, Raub TJ, Bazer FW. Role of uteroferrin in transplacental iron transport in the pig. Fed Proc. 19;45(10):2513-8. PMID: 3527760.

[77] Ellenberger C, Wilsher S, Allen WR, Hoffmann C, Kölling M, Bazer FW, Klug J, Schoon D, Schoon HA. Immunolocalisation of the uterine secretory proteins uterocalin, uteroferrin and uteroglobin in the mare's uterus and placenta throughout pregnancy. Theriogenology. 2008 Sep 15;70(5):746-757. doi: 10.1016/j. theriogenology.2008.04.050.

[78] Miele L, Cordella-Miele E, Facchiano A, Mukherjee AB. Inhibition of phospholipase A2 by uteroglobin and antiflammin peptides. Adv Exp Med Biol. 1990;279:137-160. doi: 10.1007/978-1-4613-0651-1_9.

[79] Inpanbutr N, Miller EK, Petroff BK, Iacopino AM. CaBP9K levels during the luteal and follicular phases of the estrous cycle in the bovine uterus. Biol Reprod. 1994 Mar;50(3):561-571. doi: 10.1095/biolreprod50.3.561.

[80] Ellenberger C, Wilsher S, Allen WR, Hoffmann C, Kölling M, Bazer FW, Klug J, Schoon D, Schoon HA. Immunolocalisation of the uterine secretory proteins uterocalin, uteroferrin and uteroglobin in the mare's uterus and placenta throughout pregnancy. Theriogenology. 2008 Sep 15;70(5):746-757. doi: 10.1016/j. theriogenology.2008.04.050.

[81] Hoffman C. Morphologisch-funktionelle Untersuchungen zur Pathogenese der equinen Endometrose unter besonderer Berücksichtigung endometrialer Proteine und Kohlenhydrate[dissertation vet. med.]. 2006. Leipzig.

[82] Lehmann J, Ellenberger C, Hoffmann C, Bazer FW, Klug J, Allen WR, Sieme H, Schoon HA. Morpho-functional studies regarding the fertility prognosis of mares suffering from equine endometriosis. Theriogenology. 2011;76(7):1326-1336. doi: 10.1016/j.theriogenology.2011.06.001.

[83] Hoffman C. Morphologisch-funktionelle Untersuchungen zur Pathogenese der equinen Endometrose unter besonderer Berücksichtigung endometrialer Proteine und Kohlenhydrate[dissertation vet. med.]. 2006. Leipzig.

[84] Lehmann J, Ellenberger C, Hoffmann C, Bazer FW, Klug J, Allen WR, Sieme H, Schoon HA. Morpho-functional studies regarding the fertility prognosis of mares suffering from equine endometriosis. Theriogenology. 2011;76(7):1326-1336. doi: 10.1016/j.theriogenology.2011.06.001.

[85] Hoffman C. Morphologisch-funktionelle Untersuchungen zur

Pathogenese der equinen Endometrose unter besonderer Berücksichtigung endometrialer Proteine und Kohlenhydrate[dissertation vet. med.]. 2006. Leipzig.

[86] Lehmann J, Ellenberger C, Hoffmann C, Bazer FW, Klug J, Allen WR, Sieme H, Schoon HA. Morpho-functional studies regarding the fertility prognosis of mares suffering from equine endometriosis. Theriogenology. 2011;76(7):1326-1336. doi: 10.1016/j.theriogenology.2011.06.001.

[87] Lehmann J, Ellenberger C, Hoffmann C, Bazer FW, Klug J, Allen WR, Sieme H, Schoon HA. Morpho-functional studies regarding the fertility prognosis of mares suffering from equine endometriosis. Theriogenology. 2011;76(7):1326-1336. doi: 10.1016/j.theriogenology.2011.06.001.

[88] Aresu L, Benali S, Giannuzzi D, Mantovani R, Castagnaro M, Falomo ME. The role of inflammation and matrix metalloproteinases in equine endometriosis. J Vet Sci. 2012;13(2):171-177. doi:10.4142/jvs.2012.13.2.171

[89] Chen J, Khalil RA. Matrix Metalloproteinases in Normal Pregnancy and Preeclampsia. Prog Mol Biol Transl Sci. 2017;148:87-165. doi:10.1016/bs.pmbts.2017.04.001

[90] Aresu L, Benali S, Giannuzzi D, Mantovani R, Castagnaro M, Falomo ME. The role of inflammation and matrix metalloproteinases in equine endometriosis. J Vet Sci. 2012;13(2):171-177. doi:10.4142/jvs.2012.13.2.171

[91] Aresu L, Benali S, Giannuzzi D, Mantovani R, Castagnaro M, Falomo ME. The role of inflammation and matrix metalloproteinases in equine endometriosis. J Vet Sci. 2012;13(2):171-177. DOI:10.4142/jvs.2012.13.2.171

[92] McCawley LJ, Matrisian LM. Matrix metalloproteinases: they're not just for matrix anymore! Curr Opin Cell Biol. 2001 Oct;13(5):534-540. DOI: 10.1016/s0955-0674(00)00248-9.

[93] Hoffmann C, Ellenberger C, Mattos RC, Aupperle H, Dhein S, Stief B, Schoon HA. The equine endometriosis: new insights into the pathogenesis. Anim Reprod Sci. 2009;111: 261– 278 DOI:10.1016/j.anireprosci.2008.03.019.

[94] Hoffmann C, Ellenberger C, Mattos RC, Aupperle H, Dhein S, Stief B, Schoon HA. The equine endometriosis: new insights into the pathogenesis. Anim Reprod Sci. 2009;111: 261– 278 DOI:10.1016/j.anireprosci.2008.03.019.

[95] Chu MC, Mor G, Lim C, Zheng W, Parkash V, Schwartz PE. Low-grade endometrial stromal sarcoma: hormonal aspects. Gynecol Oncol. 2003 Jul;90(1):170-176. doi: 10.1016/s0090-8258(03)00258-0

[96] Schöniger S, Schoon HA. The Healthy and Diseased Equine Endometrium: A Review of Morphological Features and Molecular Analyses. Animals (Basel). 2020;10(4):625. DOI:10.3390/ani10040625

[97] Schöniger S, Schoon HA. The Healthy and Diseased Equine Endometrium: A Review of Morphological Features and Molecular Analyses. Animals (Basel). 2020;10(4):625. DOI:10.3390/ani10040625

[98] Hoffmann C, Ellenberger C, Mattos RC, Aupperle H, Dhein S, Stief B, Schoon HA. The equine endometriosis: new insights into the pathogenesis. Anim Reprod Sci. 2009;111: 261– 278. DOI:10.1016/j.anireprosci.2008.03.019.

[99] Hoffmann C, Ellenberger C, Mattos RC, Aupperle H, Dhein S, Stief B, Schoon HA. The equine

endometriosis: new insights into the pathogenesis. Anim Reprod Sci. 2009;111: 261– 278. DOI:10.1016/j. anireprosci.2008.03.019.

[100] Streuli CH, Schmidhauser C, Kobrin M, Bissell MJ, Derynck R. Extracellular matrix regulates expression of the TGF-beta 1 gene. J Cell Biol. 1993;120(1):253-260. doi: 10.1083/ jcb.120.1.253.

[101] Raila G. Zur Pathogenese der Endometrose der Stute - Morphologisch-funktionelle Untersuchungen. Diss. Med. Vet. Leipzig. 2000.

[102] Border WA, Noble NA. Transforming growth factor beta in tissue fibrosis. N Engl J Med. 1994;331(19):1286-1292. doi: 10.1056/ NEJM199411103311907.

[103] Walter I, Handler J, Miller I, Aurich C. Matrix metalloproteinase 2 (MMP-2) and tissue transglutaminase (TG 2) are expressed in periglandular fibrosis in horse mares with endometriosis. Histol Histopathol. 2005;20(4):1105-13. doi: 10.14670/ HH-20.1105.

[104] Aresu L, Benali S, Giannuzzi D, Mantovani R, Castagnaro M, Falomo ME. The role of inflammation and matrix metalloproteinases in equine endometriosis. J Vet Sci. 2012;13(2):171-177. doi:10.4142/jvs.2012.13.2.171

[105] Hoffman C, Ellenberger C, Mattos RC et al.: The equine endometriosis: new insights into the pathogenesis. Animal Reproductive Science. 2009;3(2-4):261-278. DOI:10.1016/j. anireprosci.2008.03.019.

[106] Aresu L, Benali S, Giannuzzi D, Mantovani R, Castagnaro M, Falomo ME. The role of inflammation and matrix metalloproteinases in equine endometriosis. J Vet Sci. 2012;13(2):171-177. doi:10.4142/jvs.2012.13.2.171

[107] Aresu L, Benali S, Giannuzzi D, Mantovani R, Castagnaro M, Falomo ME. The role of inflammation and matrix metalloproteinases in equine endometriosis. J Vet Sci. 2012;13(2):171-177. doi:10.4142/jvs.2012.13.2.171

[108] Olman, M. Beyond TGF-β: a prostaglandin promotes fibrosis. Nat Med. 2009. 15. 1360-136. DOI: https:// doi.org/10.1038/nm1209-1360

[109] Oga T, Matsuoka T, Yao C, Nonomura K, Kitaoka S, Sakata D, Kita Y, Tanizawa K, Taguchi Y, Chin K, Mishima M, Shimizu T, Narumiya S. Prostaglandin F(2alpha) receptor signaling facilitates bleomycin-induced pulmonary fibrosis independently of transforming growth factor-beta. Nat Med. 2009;15(12):1426-1430. doi: 10.1038/nm.2066.

[110] Oga T, Matsuoka T, Yao C, Nonomura K, Kitaoka S, Sakata D, Kita Y, Tanizawa K, Taguchi Y, Chin K, Mishima M, Shimizu T, Narumiya S. Prostaglandin F(2alpha) receptor signaling facilitates bleomycin-induced pulmonary fibrosis independently of transforming growth factor-beta. Nat Med. 2009;15(12):1426-1430. doi: 10.1038/nm.2066.

[111] Jabbour HN, Sales KJ, Smith OP, Battersby S, Boddy SC. Prostaglandin receptors are mediators of vascular function in endometrial pathologies. Mol Cell Endocrinol. 2006;252(1-2):191-200. doi: 10.1016/j.mce.2006.03.025.

[112] Szóstek AZ, Siemieniuch MJ, Lukasik K, Galvão AM, Ferreira-Dias GM, Skarzynski DJ. mRNA transcription of prostaglandin synthases and their products in the equine endometrium in the course of fibrosis. Theriogenology. 2012 Sep 1;78(4):768-776. doi: 10.1016/j. theriogenology.2012.03.024.

[113] Rebordão MR, Amaral A, Lukasik K, Szóstek-Mioduchowska A,

Pinto-Bravo P, Galvão A, Skarzynski DJ, Ferreira-Dias G. Impairment of the antifibrotic prostaglandin E2 pathway may influence neutrophil extracellular traps-induced fibrosis in the mare endometrium. Domest Anim Endocrinol. 2019;67:1-10. doi: 10.1016/j.domaniend.2018.10.004.

[114] Rebordão MR, Amaral A, Lukasik K, Szóstek-Mioduchowska A, Pinto-Bravo P, Galvão A, Skarzynski DJ, Ferreira-Dias G. Impairment of the antifibrotic prostaglandin E2 pathway may influence neutrophil extracellular traps-induced fibrosis in the mare endometrium. Domest Anim Endocrinol. 2019;67:1-10. doi: 10.1016/j.domaniend.2018.10.004.

[115] Hoffman C, Ellenberger C, Mattos RC et al.: The equine endometriosis: new insights into the pathogenesis. Animal Reproductive Science. 2009;3(2-4): 261-278. DOI:10.1016/j.anireprosci.2008.03.019.

[116] Hoffman C, Ellenberger C, Mattos RC et al.: The equine endometriosis: new insights into the pathogenesis. Animal Reproductive Science. 2009;3(2-4): 261-278. DOI:10.1016/j.anireprosci.2008.03.019.

[117] Rebordão MR, Amaral A, Lukasik K, Szóstek-Mioduchowska A, Pinto-Bravo P, Galvão A, Skarzynski DJ, Ferreira-Dias G. Impairment of the antifibrotic prostaglandin E2 pathway may influence neutrophil extracellular traps-induced fibrosis in the mare endometrium. Domest Anim Endocrinol. 2019;67:1-10. doi: 10.1016/j.domaniend.2018.10.004.

[118] Dascanio JJ, McCue PM, editors. Equine Reproductive Procedures. 1st ed. Chichester: Wiley;2014. 68 p. DOI: 10.1002/9781118904398

[119] Keller A, Neves AP, Aupperle H, et al. Repetitive experimental bacterial infections do not affect the degree of uterine degeneration in the mare. Anim Reprod Sci. 2006.94:276-279

[120] Allen, W.R. (1993), Proceedings of the John P. Hughes International Workshop on Equine Endometritis. Equine Veterinary Journal, 25: 184-193. https://doi.org/10.1111/j.2042-3306.1993.tb02940.x

[121] Dascanio JJ, McCue PM, editors. Equine Reproductive Procedures. 1st ed. Chichester: Wiley;2014. 102 p. DOI: 10.1002/9781118904398